Praise for *Experiencing Infertility*

"This outstanding book deserves to be read by clients and therapists worldwide."
—Jan Silverman, MSW, American Society of Reproductive Medicine,
Mental Health Professional Group Newsletter

"This book is written from the heart. . . . An excellent and compassionate companion for couples struggling with infertility."
—J. C. Guerra, M.D., founder of baby-care.com

"The single best book on coping with the emotional aspect of infertility that I've ever read. As you read, you quickly realize that the authors actually 'get it' . . . that they truly uderstand what it is like to experience infertility."
—Frencesca Lindquist, director of community services, Child of My Dreams.com

"Peoples and Rovner-Ferguson sensitively ask the questions that have been on all our minds and provide compassionate answers to help couples move through what they have identified as the four states of infertility: crisis, acceptance, resolution, and epilogue."
—DES Action Newsletter

"Debby Peoples and Harriette Rovner-Ferguson faced difficult struggles with infertility; now that they've made it to the other side they've written a book to help others through the battle."
—*New York Times*

Experiencing Infertility

Experiencing Infertility

An Essential Resource

DEBBY PEOPLES, M.S.W.
and
HARRIETTE ROVNER FERGUSON, C.S.W.

W·W·NORTON & COMPANY

New York   London

First published under the title *What to Expect When You're Experiencing Infertility*

The information we offer in this book is not intended as a replacement for psychotherapy. Readers who are in excessive emotional pain should consult with a licensed mental health provider.

For Psalm 139: 7–10: Scripture taken from *The Holy Bible, New International Version,* © 1973, 1978, 1984 The International Bible Society. Used by permission of Zondervan Bible Publishers.

The text of this book is composed in Bembo
with the display set in Bembo
Composition and manufacturing by The Haddon Craftsmen, Inc.
Book design by Jacques Chazaud

Library of Congress Cataloging-in-Publication Data

Peoples, Debby.
What to expect when you're experiencing infertility : how to cope with the emotional crisis and survive it / Debby Peoples and Harriette Rovner Ferguson.
p.   cm.
Includes bibliographical references and index.
ISBN 0-393-04104-2
1. Infertility—Psychological aspects. I. Ferguson, Harriette Rovner. II. Title.
RC889.P36   1998
616.6'92'0019—dc21   97-42847
                                                          CIP

ISBN 0-393-32000-6 pbk.

W. W. Norton & Company, Inc., 500 Fifth Avenue, New York, N.Y. 10110
www.wwnorton.com

W. W. Norton & Company Ltd., 10 Coptic Street, London WC1A 1PU

1 2 3 4 5 6 7 8 9 0

To
Matthew, Evan, and Brian,
Florence and William,
Selma, Mary,
and Joyce:

with all my love—Debby

To
Fred, Tessa, and Taylor:

Thank you from the bottom of my heart—Harriette

ACKNOWLEDGMENTS

This book has its roots in a friendship born of a mutual dream. But to become a reality, a dream must be supported and nurtured by others. With deep-felt appreciation for helping us reach our dream, we sincerely thank the following people:

HEIDE LANGE, our agent, for believing in this project and in us from the beginning;

JILL BIALOSKY, our editor, for understanding our need to share this information;

HY FRANKEL, for encouraging us to forge ahead and never doubting this work should be published;

CHARLOTTE SHEEDY, for giving us our initial words of encouragement;

DR. ELLEN MILLER, for reviewing our medical information;

KATHY JOHNSON and DOROTHY GROSSKOPF, for creating a powerful witches' brew of wisdom and inspiration;

SUSAN BERG, MAUREEN BOYLE, ALLA BOZARTH, AARON BRITVAN, PEGGY BRUHN, DOMINIC and TERESA CANDIDO, FATHER PAUL COSTELLO, ALICE DOMAR, REV. CHARLES DREW, DAVID ECKERT, COLEEN FRIEDMAN, SUSAN GARDNER, SUZANNE GLYNN, RABBI BRUCE GREENBAUM, RANDI GUGGENHEIMER, BARBARA HILL, CANDACE HURLEY, IRA KALINA, ROBERT and SYBIL LEFFERTS, REV. KATE LEHMAN, JOYCE MAGID, SUSAN MORLEY, NANCY NEWMAN, REV. JOANNE OWENS, REV. KEN PAGE, HARRY RIECKELMAN, LINDA SALZER, SHERYL STERN, ALEXANDRA STODDARD, DR. FRAN TANEY, and FATHER MICHAEL VITRANO, for so willingly sharing their knowledge and contributing to the creation of our book;

TRACY PRICE and SUSAN NOBLE, for their assistance in organizing the information in this book;

GERI LIPSHULTZ, JUDE TREDER-WOLFF, and DEBORAH ZELIZER, for inspiring our creativity;

JANE ALTER and DENISE BROESLER, for supplying us with *RESOLVE* newsletters;
BARBARA BONEILLO, SUSAN BONGIORNO, LAURA CASSELL, CAROL DENBY, DEB-
    ORAH EDWARDS, JAN FINE, MELODY FLOYD, SUSAN GARDNER, BARBARA
    HEARNE, SONIA HIEGER, PEGGY RICHARDSON, CAROLYN SCANLON, MICHAEL
    SHANK, BONITA VALEZ, WENDY VOLLMUTH, LIZ WESTERMAN, and LISA
    ZOLLINGER, for reviewing and discussing our work with us;
the WAITRESSES AT FRIENDLY'S IN SMITHTOWN, for supplying us with tea, bagels,
    and smiles;
and finally, RESOLVE OF LONG ISLAND and ALL THE WOMEN AND MEN EXPERI-
    ENCING INFERTILITY, for so openly sharing their heart-warming stories with us
    and for contributing to the insights we offer in this book.

Over the years we have gathered facts, insights, and anecdotal information
from many sources, which have become integrated into our personal body of
knowledge about infertility. If we have failed to acknowledge your input into the
information in this book, please forgive us.

DEBBY'S ACKNOWLEDGMENTS

Throughout the writing of this book I have never been alone at my computer. Surrounding me always were those I hold most dear to my heart. Their support of my
dream has been a gift to be forever cherished. For accompanying me on this journey, I wish to thank first and foremost my husband, Matthew, for his love, encouragement, and the opportunity to share all that we learned during the many years
we struggled to become a family.

Evan and Brian, how much you have taught me about life and love, family and
motherhood. Your deliveries took six years (quite a long labor!), but you have
brought into my life a special light that shines in my heart and inspires me to help
others find their own happy endings.

I must thank my family, whose guidance and love have followed me through
my life: Florence and William Beitch, Lisa Zollinger, and Charles and Masha
Beitch—and of course my grandmother, Selma Gordon, who knew I was a writer
long before I did and whose encouragement and insights have enriched my life im-
measurably.

My special love, thanks, and admiration go to Joyce Magid, who has guided
me for many years with love, commitment, understanding, and patience. In your
hands I have learned to listen to my heart, write from my soul, and go after my
dreams. You will remain in my heart forever.

A particular thank you goes to Colleen Scialabba, whose mutual search for motherhood led us to friendship, understanding, laughter, and joy.

I thank my friends who have given me long breaks of laughter and caring support through the years: the members of the writer's group at the Women's Center of Huntington; Barbara and Joe Boneillo; Karen and Jim Fontana; Chris and Kathie Rutkowski; and the Great River Playgroup (Wendy, Tom, Carolyn, Kerry, Lorraine, Tony, Barbara, Kevin, Josie, Rick, Stacy, Bobby, and all the kids).

Thanks also go to Carolyn Scanlon and Laura DeNapoli, for watching my boys and keeping them safe so I could become a writer.

Thanks and love go to my friend and coauthor, Harriette Rovner Ferguson, an incredible woman with remarkable gifts and a truly loving heart. I have been blessed to have shared the experience of writing with you, and will always be grateful for the magic that brought us together.

HARRIETTE'S ACKNOWLEDGMENTS

One night while I was reading my children *The Lorax* by Dr. Seuss, I came across an ingenious word only he could create: the verb "to bigger." Finally, I found a word that described the feeling of being filled with an incredible amount of love, encouragement, and warmth. I wish to express my gratitude to all who "biggered" me as I wrote this book.

I thank my husband Fred, who found his way into my heart many years ago and whose love continues to stay there as we make our way into the future. His tireless commitment to me and our children has allowed for much that I treasure in my life.

From the deepest parts of my soul, I give thanks for my children, Tessa and Taylor. They are my greatest blessings, teachers, and inspiration. I hope as they read through this book they will find that my love underscores every line.

I will be forever grateful to Iris, Norma, Mary, Jack, Ricki, Marc, Barry, and Michael. Their constant love, devotion, encouragement, and support have given me the courage to take risks and to follow my dreams. It has been easy for me to encourage people to believe that out of darkness comes light because I come from and married into a family of survivors.

I thank Debbie Edwards and Carol Denby for being my trusted and understanding friends. Their selfless love for me and my children provided the security and freedom I needed to write. I also thank Sundarii for freely sharing her heart and home with me so I could have a quiet and loving place to create this book. I treasure their support and encouragement and our life of sisterhood.

I thank Robert and Sybil Lefferts for becoming my mentors. Their wisdom, enthusiasm, and energy for life will always be a guiding force.

A special thanks goes to Lee Kaplan for her insight and warmth, for encouraging me to reach deep inside and follow my heart, no matter what.

It is true that the friends we make as adults become our chosen family. I am truly blessed to have the Covitzes, Denbys, Edwardses, Leffertses, Marinellis, Peopleses, and Stewarts as my "family."

I am grateful for the opportunity to have witnessed the enduring wisdom and strength of my clients and members of RESOLVE of Long Island as they found their way through the crisis of infertility. They became the inspiration behind this book.

Finally I thank Debby Peoples, who I believed at the beginning of this project would be a respectful, responsible, and creative writing partner and who in the end became my magical, deep, and trusting sister. I will be eternally thankful for finding this woman who "biggers" me.

CONTENTS

III.   RESOLUTION

IV.   EPILOGUE   *209*

V.   TREATING INFERTILITY:
A Guide for Professionals   *213*

FOREWORD

ALICE D. DOMAR, PH.D.
Director, Mind/Body Center for Women's Health
Mind/Body Medical Institute
Beth Israel Deaconess Medical Center
Assistant Professor of Medicine, Harvard Medical School

"Everyone in my life, including my husband, thinks that I am a woman possessed by my drive to have a baby. I feel like a freak. Why am I responding to infertility in such a deranged way?" I have heard a variation of this plea thousands of times. Infertile individuals feel crazy, alone, and miserable during their quest to have a baby.

I have been running mind/body groups for infertile women for more than ten years and at the end of each group, I hear the same thing: "Wow, it was so fantastic to hear other women saying things which I was afraid to even think," or "Why didn't my doctor tell me to expect this kind of reaction to the medication? I thought I was abnormal until several other women told me they had the identical response," and "It feels like such a relief to hear that other couples are also struggling with disagreements about things like whether or not to attend parties where pregnant women will be present."

Infertility presents an enormous crisis. Women experiencing infertility have anxiety and depression levels equivalent to women with cancer, heart disease, or HIV-positive status. Yet people do not rush to support individuals struggling with infertility as they would if one were experiencing any other medical condition. Indeed, people often respond with blame-the-victim statements such as "You are trying too hard," "Just relax," "Why doesn't your doctor just try the same thing which my doctor tried since it worked for me," or "Why don't you just adopt and stop being so obsessed with getting pregnant?" The result is that most people experiencing infertility feel isolated, sad, and overwhelmed. They are also starving for information about what *is* a normal way to react to the infertility crisis, how to handle the inevitable disagreements over infertility with their spouse, and how to learn to feel better emotionally.

What to Expect When You're Experiencing Infertility supplies an informational feast for infertile individuals. Presented in a unique format, it leads the reader from the crisis phase to acceptance to resolution to the epilogue. What makes this book different, and so very relevant, is that not only does it help the reader learn about normal psychological reactions to infertility by means of wonderful question-and-answer format, but the tone is one of compassion. It is easy to *hear* not only the pain of the infertility patients asking the questions but also the personal wisdom and experience of the authors answering those questions.

Another strength is the enormous breadth covered in this book. The husband's viewpoint is included as are ways to handle well-meaning or even not so well-meaning comments and suggestions from friends and family. Issues of pregnancy loss, adoptive loss, and multifetal reduction are explored. Coping tools are included, such as ways for couples to communicate more effectively about infertility, how to react when a baby shower invitation arrives in the mail, and basic relaxation exercises. The book covers the whole infertility process, ranging from coping with the label of infertility, to handling the disappointment when high-tech treatment fails, to exploring options such as adoption or child-free living.

Infertile individuals feel that infertility is not only about uncomfortable and difficult procedures and treatments or feeling so alone when surrounded by fertile family and friends; it is also a constant struggle to obtain and understand complex, occasionally contradictory information. *What to Expect When You're Experiencing Infertility* can help relieve some of the psychological pain by helping the reader see that these feelings are normal, learn how to obtain support from loved ones, and cope with such a challenging and potentially traumatizing time.

PROLOGUE

I remember that day that I no longer noticed the antiseptic smell of the room or the conversation that floated out in the hallway only a few inches from where I stood. The sadness that filled my eyes made it almost impossible for me to see. I could no longer feel my hands as they rolled the stiff sheet of white paper into a ball between my fingers and stuffed it into the cold metal garbage can.

I moved so slowly then, dressing by instinct instead of attention and wrapping my thoughts in the scene that had just transpired. I replayed the doctor's apologizing eyes, the pain he left inside me from his examination, and the disjointed words from our conversation. I had heard so many others like it, offering hope and no results. That day was different—the conversation broke something inside me, snapped my resistance, went beyond my level of tolerance. I drove home without the memory of having written a check, leaving his office, or walking to my car. The exit signs of the highway served only as a replacement for a sense of direction that seemed to have failed me long ago, not as signs to be read to judge my distance from home. Distance implies space and time, a linear realm of rational units and defined order that I no longer could allow myself to be a part of. Such recognition would have been too painful a reminder for me of how much of my life had passed by, how much I had given over and away for my dream of having a baby. My dream of co-creating with God, my husband, nature, and all the forces that be. This dream had fallen away. It was beyond the realm of human control and understanding. I knew at that point that I needed help, that I could no longer do this alone.

These are the words of one woman's story. Yet, they resonated with truth in our own hearts and echoed the voices of the hundreds of men and women who have spoken with us over the past ten years. She reminded us so much of our own infertility experience; the frustrating days of doctors' appointments, specialized clinics, fertility drugs, and the losses we had endured. . . . It didn't matter that we knew how to access good health care or that we had training in communications and social work. Nothing prepared us for the emotional, physical, and financial upheaval that infertility created in our lives. We were drained, brought to our knees, and rocked to our very core—All in the pursuit of a baby and the family we had dreamed of creating since we were young girls.

Like this woman's description, there was a day when we, too, realized we needed support. For help we reached out to our family and friends. But as hard as they tried, there was little they could do. They didn't understand how the seemingly simple act of creating life could become the most complicated and involved endeavor of our lives. So we turned to self-help organizations like RESOLVE.★ There we found that with patience, understanding, and support we could make it through. We could get our sense of direction back and find a way to create the family we longed for.

It took time, but eventually we were blessed with the children we dreamed of. Now, years later, we can honestly tell you that you can survive. You will find a way out.

Carl Jung, a renowned Swiss psychiatrist, spoke of "wounded healers." He described them as people who have been through a grievous experience and lost a dream but have come out the other side, stronger and able to create a different dream. These people want to share their understanding, experiences, and learnings with others. As wounded healers we offer you this book of questions† and answers so that you will have a place to turn to when you need direction and understanding, a way to make it through a day, month, even year in your experience with infertility.

★ RESOLVE is a national nonprofit organization whose mission is to provide support and information to people experiencing infertility. See Appendix II for further information.

† The questions are edited versions of stories told to us by hundreds of infertile men and women struggling through this crisis.

INTRODUCTION

C.A.R.E.—crisis, acceptance, resolution, and epilogue: As you move through your struggle with infertility, you will find that your experiences most likely mirror these stages.

We have divided the main body of the book into four parts, one for each of the C.A.R.E. stages.★ In the *crisis* portion (Part I) we address the concerns of couples just beginning their infertility journey. As they realize they have lost the dream of easily conceiving, feelings of denial and confusion surface. (How can this be happening to me?) Their disbelief and shock increases with every passing month. Eventually couples turn to the medical community for help. Now they need to cope with the overwhelming amount of critical information they receive from doctors, nurses, and lab technicians, all of whom offer hopeful treatments for fulfilling their dream. As couples listen, often following the recommended course of

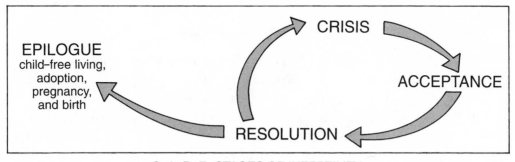

C. A. R. E. STAGES OF INFERTILITY

★ We have also included a section for professionals (Part V) along with a self-help guide (Appendix I) and a resource directory listing the addresses and phone numbers of organizations that deal with infertility (Appendix II).

treatments, they pray the procedures will work. If a cure is not found within a tolerable amount of time, everything changes as infertility becomes a lifestyle. Patients begin to see the world from a different perspective: a simple trip to the mall or an invitation to a family gathering can become reminders of their lost dream.

In time, the grueling nature of infertility moves all couples to a level of *acceptance*. In Part II we answer the questions infertile couples have when they accept their reality and begin to make major life decisions and choices. Should they pursue pregnancy and childbirth at any cost? Is the ability to parent as important as biological ties? Could they be happy living child-free?

Eventually the answer comes, suddenly for some couples, slowly for others. Either they will get pregnant and carry to term or begin moving along another path to *resolution*. In Part III we address the issues couples have while they are pregnant, waiting for a child to arrive, or settling into their commitment to live child-free. It is during this time that the future holds both the unknown and a renewed sense of hope.

Finally, when the child arrives or child-free living becomes a way of life, couples move on to the *epilogue* of their infertility story. They reconnect with the world again as they accept and integrate infertility as a permanent yet less dominant part of their identity. They are now able to comfortably look back on what they have been through and see all that has wounded them and all that they have gained.

We hope, as you read through these pages, that you will find *your* answers—not so much in our words but in the words you say to yourself. For it is there you can discover that you are not alone and not destined to live in this crisis forever.

NOTE TO PROFESSIONALS

In our desire to share the profound emotional experience of infertility patients with the professional community, we have included a substantial section specifically aimed at the mental health provider, physician, nurse, and adoption specialist. In Part V we answer questions from health-care providers to show how reactions such as depression and anxiety, once considered pathological, are actually normal responses to the crisis of infertility. In addition to our own research, we have also included how-to's, guidelines, and techniques recommended by numerous other professionals in the field. It is our hope that this information will give you a comprehensive look at the infertility experience from the inside out and will provide you with new insights and understanding into the challenges faced by infertile couples.

I

—

CRISIS

1

Who Am I?
Infertility and Identity

For men and women the experience of infertility is so dissimilar, it is hard to believe that the same word, "infertile," could apply to both genders. The way infertility affects a woman's identity, how she deals with her feelings, and even how society deals with her are quite different from the way a man moves through this same crisis.

Aware of this fact, we felt it necessary to divide our introductory comments and subsequent questions by gender. However, it is our hope that both men and women will read the chapter in its entirety to reach a greater understanding about the impact infertility has on male and female identity.

WOMEN AND INFERTILITY

As she looked at the woman in the mirror, her body grew warm. She didn't recognize the face that now stared back at her. What is happening to me? Why am I so different from other women? What is wrong with me? Please help me, she called out to that part of herself she could no longer see.

We expect a mirror to reflect back an exact image of what stands before it. But the reality is that mirrors show us more about how we feel than how we look.

Like most of us in the throws of infertility, you may no longer recognize yourself. You *have* changed. Your quest for pregnancy has led you to a strange and unfamiliar place within yourself, one that calls so strongly it seems to have taken away all free will. Your thoughts, actions, and energy all go toward getting that baby, who is going to "fix" everything. The baby who will tell you you are normal, seal the love between you and your husband, give you back your rightful place in your family, and make you feel in step with the world around you. No wonder you are so scared. Your emotions are so intense. Not having this baby threatens your life, your very existence in the world. What power we place in the hands of such a tiny baby!

What is this power? What is the lure of motherhood? Certainly the answer is not the same for everyone, but we have found, both through our personal and professional experience and through our research, that the pursuit of motherhood is influenced by many factors. Certainly personal desires, the influences of family and friends, cultural pressures, and religious teachings all play an important role in the desire for and the pursuit of motherhood. Some researchers even argue that instinctual forces pull on women as well.

But perhaps the most profound reason for wanting to become a mother is the desire most women have, either consciously or unconsciously, to be "like" and/or "better" than their own mothers. In her book *Finding Herself,* Ruthellen Josselson talks about the mother/daughter connection as it relates to identity. "To the little girl, being liked means being like. Attachment implies sameness. 'I love my mother and want to grow up to be just like her' is the hallmark of identification processes in the little girl. With becoming like mother and therefore pleasing her comes the assurance of remaining forever attached to her."[1] Even those who reject their mothers may be drawn to motherhood in an effort to fix or mend the relationship. By doing a better job with their own children they believe they get a second chance.

Because this identification with mother is an integral part of a woman's self-image, not being able to identify because of infertility means for many, not being able to identify with any woman. This disconnection from gender leaves in its wake a harrowing state of psychological confusion and chaos. Getting pregnant and having a baby soon become as essential as breathing.

An asthma sufferer immediately narrows her focus during each attack. Everything she does during that period of crisis will center around getting her breath back. When a woman is struggling to become a mother, just like a person struggling to breathe, nothing else matters. Her focus narrows: Some women quit their jobs, forgo their sex lives, and withdraw from family and society. Some women put off buying clothes expecting to be pregnant, and arrange their very lives around menstrual cycles, doctors' appointments, and times they must take their medications. They go into a cocoon of crisis and wait, counting the months the way other women count days. Time passes, hope dwindles, and yet the search for that baby continues.

Women who give birth to or adopt children and then lose them feel as if their own lives have been threatened. The baby you have in your mind is as real to you as any live baby. To not find that child is to lose a piece of yourself that seems critical to your existence. However, becoming a full-time infertile woman engulfed in crisis can also be unhealthy—to your body, mind, and spirit. Infertility leaves no part of you or your life untouched; it seeps into your being and becomes who you are. Left unchecked it can become all you are. Unless . . .

Unless you once again expand your vision of yourself, and learn to see beyond your infertility to the loving and caring person, wife, friend, daughter, and sister you are. To do this, you will have to acknowledge the fact that you have changed and work to integrate the old parts of yourself with the new ones.

One way to help you do this is by designing a pie chart of who you are. When you are ready, draw a circle and imagine all the different parts of yourself—the roles you play and the traits you possess. Divide the chart into pie pieces with the most important aspects being the largest. Include any new roles or traits that you have developed as a result of your infertility. Be as honest with yourself as you possibly can. The following are examples of the pie charts two women have shared with us. Looking at them may remind you of things you may have forgotten about yourself, that should be included in your own chart.

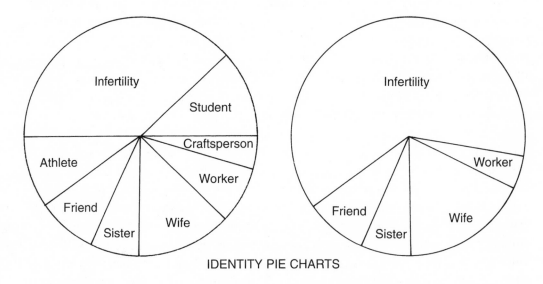

IDENTITY PIE CHARTS

Once you have finished with your chart, take a good look at it. Have you found room to be more than an infertile woman? Know that on different days of your cycle, even different months, the pie chart will most likely change. And recognize that, as you come closer to resolution the chart will change even more. The important thing to remember is that this chart may help you to see a more complete picture of yourself, the you that really exists in the mirror. It may also help you to see choices and options that perhaps you have not considered.

Being infertile may make you feel you are "less than, or not as good as." But we are here to tell you that you are no less a person, no less a woman, than anyone else. The hard lessons you learn during your search for your child will lead you to stretch your mind and heart. And someday when the crisis is over, your life will change, and you will receive the special gifts of joy and happiness that resolution can bring.

1. I'm Obsessed by Infertility

I think I'm obsessed with my infertility. I think about it all the time. Just about everywhere I go and everything I do has to do with my infertility. Going to my doctor and a support group help to keep me sane. At work I get away from it for a little while, but to be honest I usually can't wait to get home to talk to one of my infertile friends. Everyone keeps telling me to take a break, that I'm getting too crazy with all this, but I can't. Are they right? Am I too obsessed?

We haven't met a woman who *wasn't* "obsessed" with her infertility. Can you imagine anyone subjecting herself to all the medical procedures—biopsies, blood tests, hysterosalpingograms, inseminations, surgeries, and drugs—and to the roller coaster of emotions—humiliation, anger, depression, anxiety, and fear—without the kind of energy that an obsession can fuel? Can you have that kind of drive without always keeping your eye on the light at the end of the tunnel?

Think about the Olympics. Have you heard or read about the training the athletes must endure? Many of them get up at 5 A.M. to practice. Then they go to school or a part-time job, during which they no doubt spend much of their time thinking about what they can do differently or better next time. Then a short while later it's back to the gym, the track, or the pool for more hours of rigorous, painfully difficult training. Like the Olympics, trying to have a baby is a time-limited, one-shot deal. You must stay focused and attentive to your needs, determined but flexible. And just like an athlete you must plan strategies and change them when they aren't working. Everyday you work to reach your goal. When you get up in the morning, you take your temperature or use an ovulation predictor test. This is part of your training. Do you have a doctor's appointment or a blood test? Do you need to fill a perscription or buy another ovulation predictor test? You have to plan your strategy.

FOCUSING

However, there might be times when your infertility thoughts truly get in the way or times when you are so exhausted from trying to keep up with the demands of treatment that you need a break, if only for a few moments. Here's an exercise to help you switch gears and think about something other than your infertility. We call this technique "focusing." It can be done while you are driving, watching television, or cooking dinner.

Let's say, for example, that you suddenly realize you have no idea what you have been watching on television because your thoughts of infertility have completely invaded your mind. You need to bring yourself back to the present. Begin by taking a deep breath. Say to yourself,

> I am sitting on the couch, the couch is being supported by the floor beneath it, my feet are on the ground, I am wearing a pair of blue jeans, a white shirt. I have my sneakers on. I am watching the television screen and I see my husband sitting next to me. He is wearing. . . .

And so on. By using this technique you regain control by simply bringing your thoughts back to the present moment.

Like an athlete training for the Olympics, you will want to include breaks in your schedule from time to time. But also remember that your obsession to beat the infertility is necessary because it keeps you going and gets you closer to your goal of creating your family.

2. Why Am I So Angry?

It seems like every time I sit down and watch TV, I end up turning it off. I can't believe how insensitive sponsors and advertisers are to people like me. All those commercials about babies and motherhood. There is one that really kills me, about the wife telling the husband that the pregnancy test was positive. They look so happy and contented with each other. After I watch that one I just want to throw the TV across the room. Then in the supermarket—oh that's the best—the tampons are in the same isle as the diapers and baby food. It makes me nuts. Sometimes I think I get too mad, but I can't seem to help it. Is it the fertility drugs or what? Are there other people out there who feel this way?[2]

Many infertile people feel as angry as you do. In fact, it has only been through hindsight and our research that we have come to better understand the anger we encountered during this time. It might help you to know more about what anger is, where it comes from, and what purpose it serves.

Perception is everything. For each of us the information we bring to every situation affects how we interpret it. When you walk into the grocery store and see the tampons next to the baby food and the diapers, you might feel as if the grocer had strategically placed these items to remind you that you are caught in between two worlds: the harsh reality of your infertility and the fantasy of someday buying baby food and diapers. Your anger builds inside.

However, that is your story. Everyone who walks down that isle brings their own story, their own information, to the experience. A woman in menopause buying baby food for her grandchild may see the tampons as a reminder of her own loss of fertility, which may invoke sad feelings for her. On the other hand, a teenager buying tampons might not even notice the baby food. The same situation that makes one person angry may not affect another person at all, and may make still another person sad. As you can see, not one of these responses is inherently right or wrong.

But your anger is not just a response to the psychological pressures of infertility. It may also have a biochemical component to it, prompted by the use of fertility drugs. The effect may be an increase in your normal or typical angry reaction to a level that feels exaggerated or uncomfortable. Many women have reported this to their doctors. However, not every doctor supports this theory. As one woman told us,

> When I told my doctor I was not feeling like myself, that I was much angrier than usual, his reaction was that it wasn't the drugs, it was me. He then proceeded to give me the name and phone number of the hospital social worker. It wasn't till I spoke with other women that I found out that they were having the same experience with the drug.

As women, we know that anything affecting our hormones can make us feel differently. It is logical to assume that putting high doses of hormones into our bodies will also affect us. Infertility drugs have made some women release five, ten, twelve, or more eggs at one time. It doesn't seem likely that a woman's body could work in overdrive like that without having a reaction.

It is important, however, to remember that, while these hormones may be linked to the intensity of your reactions, they are not the sole determinant of anger. "Your cognitive awareness and interpretation of an emotion-provoking event or situation is a second, equally important component."[3] Therefore even if you could somehow rid yourself of the chemical portion of your anger, your infertility would still make you feel angry at times. Since you are "stuck" with this anger, perhaps it would be helpful to see its positive aspects.

In their book *When Anger Hurts*, Matthew McKay, Peter D. Rogers, and Judith McKay state that *anger stops stress "by discharging or blocking awareness of painful levels of emotional or physical arousal.*"[4] Thus anger can actually protect you against an onslaught of unmanageable and sometimes inappropriate emotions. For example, instead of experiencing deep sadness in the middle of the supermarket and expressing it by crying, you get angry. You might find that letting anger out can also relieve some muscle tension and frustration, and can serve as a defense in a physically or psychologically threatening situation.

But while anger can protect, it can also feel so bad at times that you may find yourself needing to release it. What should you do with all this anger? Some of the techniques given in the "Self-Help Guide" (Appendix I), such as the relaxation, visualization, and the writing exercises, may help you to reduce anger and stress. In addition, some people find crying, physical exercise, and hard work good ways to handle anger. Still others work on their anger by talking with friends, going to a support group, or seeing a therapist. No matter what method you choose, try to remember that, like many things in life, anger is a double-edged sword which, when kept in perspective, can be used to your best advantage.

3. I Really Think I'm Going Nuts!

I've basically gotten most everything I have wanted in my life. I've worked hard for it, and I've achieved a lot. I am an architect for a large corporation. My husband and I have a good relationship. We live in a beautiful apartment in the city and have a weekend home in the country. We have the kind of life I've always dreamed of having. It took us a while to make the decision to have a family, but when we finally did, I wanted it very badly. But, for the first time, no matter what I do, no matter how hard I try, no matter how well I follow the rules, I can't seem to get pregnant.

After two years I decided I could not wait any longer so I made all the right contacts with excellent physicians and went through the tests, drugs, and so on. But they still haven't diagnosed our problem, and are calling it, "unexplained infertility." You'd think that by this point I would have learned my lesson and not get my hopes up every month. But I do, I can't help myself. Every little twinge in my abdomen or wave of nausea makes me believe that this could be the month.

Each time my period comes, I feel so incredibly let down. I am doing all these crazy things too, especially around the time I am expecting to start my period. Like last month, I made a deal with myself that I wouldn't buy a great pair of jeans I wanted because if I bought them, that would mean that I wasn't pregnant. If I didn't get them, then I would be. How stupid can you get? Of course I got my period and I didn't get the jeans.

I also look to see if God is sending me any signs about whether or not this is the month I will get pregnant. Like if it's a rainy or ugly day, I think. He's telling me that the outcome will not be good. I really think I am going nuts. Am I the only one running around with these crazy thoughts and feeling so bad?

Like you, many people were raised with the notion that if you work hard enough and play by the rules, then you will be able to get anything you want. Unfortunately the truth is that we do not have 100 percent direct control over birth, death, health, or reproduction. It is this lack of control that is usually the most difficult to deal with while coping with infertility, especially for people like you who have made this work ethic an integral part of who you are.

You have achieved a lot of success in your life. Having a baby "should" have been easy, and even if not easy, working hard "should" have gotten you what you wanted. But infertility doesn't work that way. Your beliefs, self-esteem, fulfillment from work, relationships—everything you know has been challenged, leaving you both sad and scrambling to make some kind of sense out of what is happening. So how do you reconcile what there is no explanation for and still live with it?

Many people begin to use belief systems that they normally would not adhere to. Not buying those jeans made you believe it would signal a pregnancy. Although this way of thinking may be new to you, employing what some might consider "superstitious" beliefs is a way of coping. These thoughts may feel crazy, but it is not you or your behavior that is crazy; it is the situation. Your infertility has defied all the rules you believed to be true, and you are desperately searching for new ones.

It may surprise you to know that the vast majority of women we have spoken to have used similar tactics when dealing with their infertility. Women put off buying clothes, changing jobs, going on vacation, and even buying tampons in the hope that such decisions will somehow improve their chances for pregnancy. Even though we all know that avoiding a purchase will not make you any more fertile, most of us have at one time or anther taken comfort in such a thought.

If this new belief system fails often enough, however, most people begin to look to other ways of coping with a crisis. For some, this means turning to prayer, religion, God, a higher power, or to New Age beliefs. Many people see religion as a way to deal with those things that we as humans cannot control or explain. Turning to one's faith can be the first step in making the shift from thought and action toward an acceptance of life's circumstances. "For many people, acceptance and spiritual enlightenment are one and the same."[5] (See Chapter 8 for a more thorough discussion on religion.)

However, it is important to recognize that acceptance does not mean giving up. In fact the opposite is true. When the burden of what you cannot control is lifted from your shoulders, you can see more clearly and direct your energy toward productive efforts that can help you reach your goal.

This means separating your "doing" self, the part of you that makes things happen—from your "spiritual" self, the part able to trust that, one way or another, things will work out, even if not as originally planned. Your doing self will get you to your doctor appointments and read the latest books on treatments. Your spiritual self will help find peace while you wait for direction, answers, and peace. It will send you to the doctor month after month even when your doing self says, "What's the point?" It's the part of you connected to your heart and to hope. It is the part of you that learns that the path to your dreams is not always within your control, that sometimes you get what you want in ways you never expected.

4. I'm Not Attractive Anymore

Infertility has robbed me of so much, but now it's starting to affect the way I feel about making love with my husband. I know I'm not attractive anymore, let alone sexy. Lately whenever he approaches me to have sex, I find a reason why I can't. We had a great sex life before all of this, and now I am truly not interested. I feel lousy about this. *Help!*

You've been poked and probed by the doctor in the morning, you keep a temperature chart and thermometer on the nightstand, the ovulation predictor test is in the bathroom, needles are in the medicine cabinet, pregnant women are everywhere, and you are bloated from infertility drugs. Is it really a surprise that your sex life is not what it used to be?

All infertility patients think they should be able to split their feelings about their body into two worlds: one for infertility and one for intimacy. Unfortunately this isn't easy. Even couples who have moved on to high-tech treatment in which sex is no longer a prerequisite in their baby-making process find that sex and reproduction are inextricably linked.

If sex were purely a physical act, you would likely have no problem making love with your husband. But as a women you bring not only your body to the bedroom, but also your feelings about who you are. Believing that you are no longer attractive is one sign that your feelings about who you are have changed. This is a common experience for women who are going through infertility. Many women report feeling like "less of a woman" and often project these feelings onto their husbands, assuming they feel the same. This is not really so surprising, when you consider that we often see ourselves differently from how others see us. We look at ourselves with a very subjective, scrutinizing eye. As one woman told us,

> I realized in the course of a two-day period I seemed to see two different women in the mirror. The first day—no doubt I was in a good mood—I felt really good about how I looked, pleased that everything staring back at me was just fine, just how I like it to be, taking into account that trading looks with Christy Brinkley is out of the question. Then the next day—when the bad mood had set in—I was pale, my eyes looked like they were no longer a pleasing shape, my lashes seemed to be shorter, and how in the world did my nose get bigger?

As with this woman, the state you are in now is not permanent. However, recognizing this and being able to make love are quite different. What can you do? First, we suggest a reality check with your husband. Ask him if you are, in fact less attractive to him now. Second, as much as is humanly possible, try to separate your baby making from your love making. Although this can be difficult, given the right conditions you may be able to revive that time, before your infertility, when you did feel more attractive and sexual. Here are some things that might help you get there:

1. Schedule love making for fun to a time when you cannot possibly get pregnant and when you don't have a doctor's appointment the next day. This will immediately take the pressure off.
2. Use candles, wine, a different setting, a new nightgown or negligee, sheets, anything that will not remind you of what you usually do to make a baby. For those couples who can afford it, getting away to a hotel for an evening or weekend can help to separate you even more from all the baby-making reminders.
3. Prior to making love, prepare yourself through visualization. Reenact a fantasy. Or try to remember what it was like before the infertility, back when you were dating or just married. If visualization is difficult, try talking to your husband about the "old days." Saying to him, "Remember when we used to . . . ?" may send both of you back to that time.
4. You, like many people, may benefit from watching a romantic or even an X-rated movie prior to love making. Such films can stimulate imagination and briefly take you outside of your normal world.
5. If you do notice thoughts about your struggle with infertility while you are

making love, quickly try to think of something else. Divert your attention by bringing the visualization, the movie, or anything other than your infertility to the forefront of your consciousness.

No matter what you do, try to give yourself a break. Remember, all couples experience changes in their sex lives. Even couples not experiencing infertility have found themselves wanting to make love less than when they first got married. Changes in sexual desire over time are based on many factors ranging from a crisis to something as insignificant as a busy work schedule. Your reasons are well founded and will no doubt change in time. Although the waiting can be difficult, we know that your new feelings about love making are quite common and, more often than not, temporary.

5. I'm Feeling Left Out of the Group

Every year around the holidays all the neighbors on the block get together. I dread this party because inevitably someone always asks, "So, when are you and Jim going to have a baby?" While I knew this year was going to be especially hard because we just went through our third unsuccessful IVF (*in vitro* fertilization) cycle, I never anticipated it would be unbearable. The women stood around talking about all the gifts they had brought for their children, while the men talked about the race to put together all those toys in one night. And all the while I sat there sipping my eggnog feeling like such a complete misfit. I couldn't stand that feeling. I am a very successful businesswoman, and I pride myself on my ability to talk to anyone. But this time, I was speechless.

It was so uncomfortable that I pretended to feel sick and went home an hour after we arrived. I can't wait till the day when I can go to these parties and feel like I am part of the neighborhood crowd—or any crowd for that matter. I don't know how much more of this I can take. What if I never get pregnant?

What does it mean to you to be part of a group or a neighborhood crowd? Remember back to your high school days. Did you want to be in with the cheer leaders, the athletes, the artists, the partiers, the really smart kids, or some other group? For each of us the answer will be different.

Are any of your feelings of being left out similar to the ones you had in high school? What did you do back then when you felt that way? Did you constantly try to find a way into the more desirable group? Or did you search out a group of friends who were actually more like you, who shared similar interests, concerns, and views of the world? Finding peers you were most comfortable with was really a way of protecting yourself from feeling rejected.

You can take care of yourself in exactly the same way again by focusing your attention on people whose interests and situations are more compatible with yours. In the company of other infertile women you will most likely be happier. And finding these women may not be as difficult as you might think since many infertility patients, like yourself, have turned to support organizations like RESOLVE (a national volunteer organization for those experiencing infertility.) See Appendix II for further information on this and other resources. You may find that getting through social obligations like those neighborhood parties is much easier when you know that others are waiting at home at the other end of the phone to share your stories, frustrations, and pain.

6. I Just Want to Be Normal!

My whole life I have struggled to be normal. My parents never had a lot of money, barely enough to make ends meet. I couldn't do what all the other kids could, there was no money for piano lessons or Girl Scout dues, and certainly not enough for college. So I put myself through school, and vowed that I would make a normal life for me and the family I planned on having.

I met my husband in college and got married right after graduation. We both got good jobs and saved for and bought a nice home. My plan was working perfectly until I started trying to have a baby. It took me over a year to get pregnant, and when I finally did, I ended up with an ectopic pregnancy. That was five years ago, and I haven't gotten pregnant since then.

Why is this happening to me? None of my friends have infertility problems, and no one ever had an ectopic pregnancy. They've had miscarriages but always went on to have healthy babies. I've had surgery to remove my tube, took fertility drugs, had inseminations, and still no baby.

Lately I have really been feeling envious of all my friends, so envious that I can't stand it. Whenever I talk to them I get so angry. The slightest thing will set me off. Sometimes I can't even believe what I'm saying—it doesn't feel like me at all.

I really feel like I have been dealt a bad deck of cards. I know I am lucky to have found my husband, but now I want to make a family with him. When will it be my turn to feel like everyone else?

We all know about jealousy—we don't call it the green-eyed monster for nothing. It feels terrible; we want no part of feeling jealous. But when you are infertile, there will be times that you can't help feeling you have been "dealt a bad deck of cards." And even though you are not alone in your feelings, the question remains: are you destined to stay jealous until you have the family you dream of, or is there some way to feel better until you get to feel "normal"?

Here is what one woman said about her jealous feelings:

I think the most profound shift in my own experience with jealousy came about four years into my infertility. I was really getting crazed by then. My sister had a baby, my friends had babies, everyone but me. I was jealous of them all. And then I found out my cousin was pregnant. She had what I considered at the time to be a "normal" life. She got pregnant easily, quickly, and there I sat infertile. My jealousy grew. All I could see was that here she was having this great life and mine (although in reality except for the pregnancy quite similar) was horrible. My cousin, of course, enjoyed an uneventful pregnancy: nine months of bliss, I imagined; sonograms, amnios no problem.

And then she gave birth to a baby girl with severe birth defects, problems which for whatever reason never showed up on the tests she had taken, problems which within the week would take her tiny daughter's life. My cousin's normal life, the one I had envied so, was not normal and was not one to envy anymore. After the initial shock wore off and the guilt I had over my previous feelings subsided, I began to explore for the first time exactly what it meant to be normal and why I was jealous of those I perceived who fit the bill. I needed answers.

Like this woman we both had similar experiences during our infertility that stopped us dead in our tracks and left us questioning our own definitions of a "normal" life. We hope what we learned will be helpful to you too.

We had confused the word "normal" with the word "perfect." We didn't want a normal life, we wanted a perfect life. Normal people get married, but they also get divorced. Normal people can be rich, poor, or somewhere in between. Normal people can get pregnant, and have their babies or lose their babies. And normal people can be fertile or infertile. A perfect person with a perfect life, on the other hand, would get everything she wanted when she wanted it. She would not have the kinds of problems we have had. She would not need to face difficulties, pressures, or pain. She would not live a real life, which is why perfect people with "normal" lives do not exist. They are tricks of our imagination, perhaps put there to make all of us women strive for more or for better than we have.

Even with all our imperfections, problems, and traumas, we survive. Not only do we survive, but quite often we get opportunities to grow in ways we never would have dreamed possible.

7. What If Never?

I have been married for two years, and during that time I have not been able to get pregnant. We have just started our infertility workup. I'm a little hopeful that our doctor will help us, but I can't help thinking: what if something is so wrong they won't be able to fix it?

I come from a very large family—six sisters and two brothers. As a child I played "mommies" with my sisters constantly. We would even stick pillows under our shirts to pretend we were pregnant. When I was a teenager, I babysat for our neighbors and eventually for my sister's children. I loved it. In fact I was one of the only people in our family who loved being around children. I even majored in early childhood education in college thinking I would like to spend my life being around young kids.

Now my brothers and sisters all have families, I am the only exception and I hate it. I don't know what I will do if I can't get pregnant.

When a woman chooses to become a mother, there are many reasons behind her decision. Your statement shows that many of the plans you have made for your future centered around the strong bond you have with your family and your deep desire to nurture children. Your infertility, however, has challenged these plans and is threatening your very identity.

A comparable situation would be a professional athlete waiting to see whether the knee surgery she had undergone was successful. The waiting and the uncertainty to see whether a planned-for, much-loved career would end or continue could be excruciating. Pressure to achieve the desired outcome would come from all sides: family, friends, team members, fans, and even doctors would all want to see the patient recover fully. The truth is, some patients will recover and others will not. Such is the uncertainty you now face. You are not sure whether you will be back "in the game," and it is that question that is so difficult to live with. No wonder you are so anxious to plan for the future, "just in case" things do not work out. What will happen if that critical link between bearing children and the identity you have built your life around is never made?

For most of us the answer to that question unfolds slowly, over time. It is a process of looking at family-building options and deciding which ones are right for us and which ones are not. At first, most people see only one option—pregnancy. However, if as time passes there is no pregnancy, those women who maintain a "pregnancy or nothing" view will seek out the assisted reproductive technologies or child-free living. Others who seek parenthood over pregnancy will begin to more seriously consider other options, like adoption or child-free living. This shifting can be seen in the story one woman told about her support group:

> It was clear right from the start that all the women I met were happy with their doctors and their course of treatment and said that they would never consider any of the high-tech treatments or adoption. But over time the opinions of the women began to change, and one by one they began to do many of the things they had said they would never do. Some switched doctors, some went for IVF, others inquired into surrogacy, and still others began looking into adoption.
>
> Ironically, in the end, half the group ended up adopting their children. Some decided to live without children, and some got pregnant. It was funny how things worked out. My grandmother used to tell me, "never say never." And I guess she was right because you just never know.

Most people we have met have had similar experiences. Views change over time, and people become open to other options. (We talk a lot about this shifting of views and priorities in Chapter 9). As your own medical treatment continues you will most likely find that the same thing happens to you. You will find yourself looking for new ways to create the very special family you have been longing for.

8. Sometimes I Feel Like I Want to Die

I have been infertile for the past four years. In that time we have tried everything the doctor suggested, but so far nothing has worked. I just finished my second IVF cycle, and it failed. I really don't think I will ever get pregnant, and it feels so horrible. Sometimes I feel like I want to die. All the life has been drained out of me. What is the point of my living like this?

You are in the middle of trying to cope with one of the greatest losses a woman can suffer. The closer you find yourself getting to the possibility of "never" being able to produce a biological child, the more difficult the feelings become.

Many women experiencing infertility find themselves in what feels like a chronic state of depression. Weighed down by previous losses and anticipating new ones, many infertility patients go through the motions of life, "living without living." They judge themselves by what they don't have. Unable to see joy and meaning in their lives, they begin to believe that their life is not worth living. None of the women we know who felt like they wanted to die ever acted on these thoughts, but we do believe that these feelings must always be taken seriously. Therefore it is time for appointments with two professionals: first, with your physician to rule out any medical condition that might be causing your depression, and second, with a therapist familiar with loss and grief. In encouraging you to seek help, we are not telling you that you are crazy or that there is something wrong with you. Rather, the situation you have found yourself in is feeling overwhelming to you and causing you more stress than you should have to deal with alone.

Ellen Bass and Laura Davis, in their groundbreaking book, *The Courage to Heal,* say:

> If you start feeling suicidal or compelled to hurt yourself, get help right away. Make an agreement to call a counselor or a friend if you feel you can't control your actions. Call your local suicide prevention hotline. (Find the number before you need it). . . . If the first help isn't helpful, get other help. Don't give up. When you feel bad enough to want to die, it's hard to imagine that you could ever feel any other way. But you can. And will.[6]

MEN AND INFERTILITY

You promised to take care of her on your wedding day. All "good" husbands protect their wives. Men protect their women—that's what they do. Quite a legacy to live up to, wouldn't you say? Perhaps your father protected your mother. Perhaps you saw him take on the financial responsibilities, or drive her places, or even do the discipline so she would not have to deal with things reserved for the man of the house. Even though we live in different times, you may still feel that tug from childhood that says, "take care of her, make her happy."

Today she is not happy. She looks at all the other women with their babies, goes through painful tests and treatments, moves emotionally with the flow of her cycle, and you are powerless to do anything about it. Infertility resides in the realm of the female, and all the power goes to her doctor. And so on every level you are dismissed. In most of society "if women's and men's styles are shown to be different, it is usually women who are told to change."[7] But infertility is different. Here the focus is on the women. It is the male who is told he doesn't talk about it enough, care enough, do enough. And so it is you who is accused of hiding and running—from society, testing, treatment, support groups, even from your wife.

The problem with this way of viewing infertility is that your words and actions remain misunderstood. Your ways of coping are seen as wrong. Your point of view is ignored. But how can women learn more about how you cope with infertility as a male? Samuel Osherson, in his book *Finding Our Fathers,* notes that "one obstacle to learning more about the male experience of infertility is the emotional withdrawal of men who experience fertility problems. Scientists and filmmakers often report that it is hard to find men who will talk about the experience."[8] ". . . One husband referred to [it] as the 'secret underground of men who've gone through reproductive difficulties.' "[9] Researcher Tracy MacNab, after having distributed over 500 questionnaires to better document the male experience of infertility, was able to find only fifteen men willing to participate in his research.[10]

Aline P. Zoldbrod, in her book *Men, Women and Infertility,* notes that though MacNab's work was limited in scope,

> The themes that developed from these interviews showed quite clearly that the infertility has become a major crisis [for men] after three years of active infertility struggle. Many of the upsetting feelings that their wives had been experiencing all along suddenly became understandable. Their lives began to feel out of control in general. Their self-esteem was damaged. They were distressed by the medical interventions performed on their wives' bodies. Recurrent cycles of hope and despair were experienced as various medical solutions did not work. It became painful to be around children. They resented the pressure and intrusiveness of family and friends about their plans for children. They felt socially isolated, as if they were "different from others," and afraid to talk about the infertility because others would think they were impotent. They began to grieve for the loss of their genetic line.
>
> Some men had begun to look for a higher order of meaning or spoke of the "forced examination of values" that infertility had brought about. It had taught some of them some new things about themselves. They explored their motivations for parenthood. They felt more philosophical, older, wiser, and more able to tolerate and talk about feelings.
>
> Several of the men stressed the need for a forum for men to discuss their feelings about infertility but they acknowledged how difficult it is for men to publicly address intimacy and sexuality.[11]

Although we believe men do not talk about their infertility experience because it is so upsetting for them, we also believe they do not talk or "open up" as much as women because it is not in their "nature" to do so. As John Gray says in *Men Are from Mars, Women Are from Venus,* "When a [man] Martian gets upset he never talks about what is bothering him. . . . Instead he becomes very quiet and goes to his private cave to think about his problem, mulling it over to find a solution."[12] And even if the man cannot find a solution on his own, he most times will not look to others for advice, for support, preferring nine times out of ten to stay with the problem until he can figure it out for himself. In seeking advice, some men feel less strong, less powerful, less protective of their wives.

Understanding this, we realize that opening up this book to seek information or advice meant you are truly on the look out for a solution. And as you read through this section, remember you are different from your wife. You will handle infertility from your own perspective and in your own amount of time. Recognizing the difference will leave you room for exploration, allow you to come from a place of caring and understanding toward yourself and your spouse, and will help you get to the resolution you seek.

9. I Can't Tell Them I'm Infertile

My wife and I have been having difficulty conceiving for a year. The diagnosis is male infertility. When people in my family ask us why my wife is not pregnant yet, I tell them we've been trying, and that she's seeing a specialist, but that our problem has not been diagnosed. I don't know what else to do, I can't tell them that I am infertile. Any suggestions?

Perhaps the best approach is to gain some insight into why you have been unwilling to tell the truth about your infertility thus far. In addition to not yet feeling comfortable with your diagnosis, another common reason men give for not sharing information about their infertility has to do with cultural expectations. In our culture, the mere mention of male infertility conjures up negative images of weak, frail, impotent men whose only real problem is that they don't "know how to do it right." Fertile men, on the other hand, are viewed by our society as masculine, strong, and virile—all positive, attractive images. These stereotypes, coupled with the fact that males in our culture are trained to think and act competitively, make it very difficult for men to reveal the truth about their infertility. This stigma is so pervasive that those males who do reveal their infertility problems are often subjected to offhanded comments and jokes. As a result many men will do anything they possibly can to avoid having to confront these stereotypes.

Perhaps this is also true for you: you might not be talking about your diagnosis with your family because you are trying to avoid the confrontations, comments, and stigma of being infertile. As time goes on and you and your wife begin to accept your situation, you might feel more comfortable talking about it. As one man said,

At first I didn't want to tell anyone. I even lied about my problem and blamed it on my wife. But after a while, after I had gone to enough doctors and the test results were consistent, I had no choice. I had to accept the fact that I was infertile. The thing that finally got me to talk about it was going to a RESOLVE meeting with my wife. I remember hearing these guys talk about their infertility and I would look at them and think, "they look normal."

If at some point in the future you too find yourself ready to begin discussing your infertility, you may want to choose a trusted friend or family member to confide in. Talking about your infertility is a risk, but might just be worth a try.

10. I Just Don't Care Anymore

My wife and I have been going through infertility for four years now, and to tell you the truth, I am sick of it. I don't think anything is going to work anyway, and it feels like we're just wasting money. Whenever I tell her my concerns, she tells me it's not just having a baby that I don't care about, it's everything. And as much as I hate to admit it, I think she may be right. Things that used to matter don't anymore. I used to golf and play tennis, but I'm either too tired or I just don't care anymore. I wish we would end all this infertility garbage—then I think I would be fine.

If you have endured years of being the "strong silent type"—quietly and calmly supporting your wife through her testing and treatments and the ups and downs of her cycles—then you have suffered loss after loss, just like your wife, but without anyone to talk to, share your feelings with, or even complain to. No wonder you don't care and want out. The depressive symptoms you are experiencing are most likely not just about what is happening to you now but the cumulative effect of everything from the past that has already gone wrong. So instead of just looking to quit, your best bet now is to move forward by finding a way to deal with all the losses you have endured.

The first step is to have your physician rule out any physical problems that could be contributing to your moods. Second, it may be very helpful to talk to a therapist about all that has been happening to you since your infertility began. While you may be hesitant to do so, your withdrawal from many of the people and activities you used to be involved with, while not yet serious in itself, may signal that you have had all the stress you can tolerate. A neutral professional can offer both the support and direction you may need during this difficult time and may be able to help you come to terms and make peace with the many losses you have suffered thus far.

11. I'm Hiding How I Feel

Ever since this infertility started my life is no longer my own. Everything re-volves around "her cycle." My mood's up at the beginning of the cycle and down at the end, just like my wife. The problem is, I can't tell anyone how I feel, or even complain to my wife since I always feel like I have to hide it from her. If she knew how hard this is on me, I know she would fall apart. She already thinks I want to leave her, which believe me is the last thing I want. I just want to know if other men go through this because, like I said, who would I ask?

The feelings you describe have been shared by many men and documented in the research about men's reaction to infertility. According to Zoldbrod, MacNab found that, like you, "Some husbands . . . are closely attuned to their wives' cycles of op-timism and disappointment. They are the silent partners, frightened of and em-barrassed by their own mood swings." For these husbands "a job or career does not necessarily offer protection from the feeling that life is out of control. The feelings of disappointment, inadequacy, and frustration totally pervade their lives."[13] Mac-Nab further notes, that

> men's attempt to live up to the expectation that they will face any situation without complaining or requiring support for themselves may serve initially to preserve the husband's sense of hope and maintain the energy necessary to con-tinue with life tasks through the disappointment of infertility. In the long run, however, that psychological mechanism becomes dysfunctional to men's well-being: They become socially isolated, often growing distant from their wives.[14]

A distance that is both unhealthy for the marriage and quite unnecessary. Most wives not only can *handle* hearing about their husbands' feelings but would actu-ally take comfort in knowing the truth. Knowing that you share her mood swings may help your wife to feel more secure with her own feelings and in your rela-tionship. She will no longer have to guess at what is going on for you, and will feel more comfortable approaching you with her insecurities in the future.

If you don't know where to start, or how to approach her initially with your feelings, you may want to look at Chapter 3. Techniques discussed there can help you and your wife be more open to each other's thoughts, feelings, and needs. If you do this, the crisis of infertility will do less damage and may even strengthen your marriage.

12. I Identify with My Father

Becoming a father was always very important to me. I came from a large family—there were seven of us. My father worked hard and couldn't give us much of his time, but I always looked up to him. Even though today I make probably ten times the money he makes, I still look up to him. I thought at some point, though, we would end up being more equal, like my sisters and our mother seem to be. But now that my wife hasn't been able to get pregnant, I wonder if I will ever be as good as him?

Most men set standards for themselves—of goods, bads, shoulds, and shouldn'ts—that enable them to set goals for their lives. These rules become a part of who you are, of your identity. The criteria for many of these standards are set up in early childhood and are often patterned after parents, grandparents, and/or other role models and influences. It sounds like your father was just such a role model offering you a positive, desirable view of career and fatherhood. And as long as you maintained or exceeded your father's position, you remained comfortably aligned with him. Your identity remained intact.

Infertility, however, has left you isolated from your father. You no longer are able to be "like him." The very essence of who you are and what you are about has been threatened. This experience may bring with it many feelings, but for many men none is greater than a feeling of isolation. When you talked about your sisters being more equal to your mother than you felt with your father, the picture we had in our minds was of women sharing common experiences. And while you can share with your father the similarities of work, infertility has definitely cut you off from meeting him on the intimate and common ground of fatherhood.

As Osherson states,

> a principal source of isolation for men during times of reproductive difficulty lies in the nature of their connection to other men. . . . The man may find himself confronted by his childlike yearnings for validation or approval or a moment of special connection with his own father, and he may feel as an adult . . . it is inappropriate or unsafe to talk about the confusing mix of vulnerability, hope, and disappointment that infertility brings with it. In talking with men about infer-

tility, I often have the impression that they would like to talk to their fathers about the experience more than they do, even though that wish usually goes un-acknowledged or unexpressed.[15]

Perhaps you, like many men, would like to talk to your father about some of the things you have been going through. If you can see your way clear to doing so we believe it would be a valuable experience for both of you. Since you have begun to judge your relationship with him on the fact that you are not yet a father your-self, it would be helpful to see how your own father views you and your relation-ship. Our guess is that your father already feels you are as "good" as he is. And, if he is like most parents, he probably sees you as "better" than himself in many ways.

If you cannot talk to your father about this, and we understand that many men can't, try to imagine your own grown son in this position talking to you. Step back and look at the life you have made, the things you have done and see if you would be proud of your son for doing the same things. Now think if you would judge your son harshly because he or his wife has a medical problem preventing them from having children. Would you judge him or rather feel for him? Would you wish that the problem could be solved quickly so that he and his wife could stop hurting and get on with their lives as they had planned? From this perspective the father you looked up to for so many years is probably today, not in any way, look-ing down on you but rather in his own way, hurting for you.

2

Secondary Infertility
Through the Eyes of a Parent

Here's what secondary infertility* means to everyone else:

> Secondary infertility is the inability to conceive a pregnancy or carry a pregnancy to term following the birth of one or more children. . . . Secondary infertility can and does occur among couples who earlier had little or no problem conceiving, as well as among those with a recurring infertility problem, who can be said to have experienced both primary and secondary infertility.[1]

What secondary infertility means to you:

> *Barely awake she is in the bathroom, her ovulation predictor test in hand. Fluids, sticks, and chemicals combine to forecast the coming day. When the stick turns bright blue, she awakens; thoughts race through her head: he must get to the hospital before his flight to Washington, D.C. And so she wakes her husband early, too early. "Today is the day," she tells him. "Tomorrow may be too late." He moves quickly, though reluctantly. He could live with only one child, yet he obliges.*
>
> *She will need an appointment for the insemination, and a baby-sitter, and time to pick up milk and put gas in the car. It all must go smoothly or she will blow her whole cycle—all the shots, the sonograms, and the blood tests will be for nothing. But for now she must wait for the doctor's office to open, wait to call the baby-sitter. And in this stretch of time with her husband gone and her daughter sleeping, she is filled with a hopeful anxiety. Maybe this will be the time, perhaps this is it. Just two weeks ago all hope had vanished as she bled away her desires, plans, and dreams for a second child. But today things are different again, different as they are every month when the stick turns blue and possibility plays with fate.*
>
> *The minutes of waiting feel like hours. Finally she is able to make her appointment and arrange for the baby-sitter. Her daughter sleeps soundly, perhaps too soundly, she thinks, but instead of investigating she grabs her shower and makes herself*

---

* Although women who have experienced a pregnancy loss may be considered by the medical community to have secondary infertility, the term is most commonly used to refer to those couples who have had one or more living children and are unable to conceive again. Even though there may be many medical similarities between these two groups, we recognize that the day-to-day experiences are often quite dissimilar. Therefore in this chapter we are referring to only the latter—couples who have a living child or children and who are now experiencing infertility.

ready for the day. But fate has another plan, revealed to her as her daughter awakens sweating and crying with 103-degree fever and a sore throat. And so she will spend the rest of the morning canceling her plans and making new ones. She will sit in the pediatrician's office, not in her doctor's office. And instead of hope, she will have tears, tears that will well up in her eyes as she struggles to keep her composure amid the newborns who surround her. As her emotions ride between concern for her daughter and the rage and disappointment of another month of waiting, she wonders how she will do it again. How she will get up the strength and the courage. How she will live with the guilt of giving to this invisible baby what she is told belongs to her daughter. How much longer can she wait to be pregnant, to be happy to be whole again?

Most people may know what secondary infertility is. But only couples with secondary infertility understand what this kind of nightmare feels like. Because only they must consider a third person, their child. This chapter is about the unique experience of infertility from the prospective of a parent.

From practical considerations, involving things like money and child care, to more psychological considerations, like how your child is perceiving your infertility, the experience is no longer your own. Constantly struggling to balance every decision so that it is right for you, your spouse, and your child can leave you feeling extremely pressured. And unlike other issues where you may find guidance from those who have had similar experiences, this time you will probably find yourself struggling alone for answers, with no one to turn to for advice.

This isolation is especially confusing when you consider that secondary infertility affects 1.4 million American couples.[2] So, where are these people? You know they are not at your child's school since you are the only mother or father not holding onto a toddler and a newborn. And they are not in line at the supermarket where many families have two, three, and four children tagging along. In fact, no matter where you go with your child—birthday parties, parks, libraries, wherever you cannot stop being reminded of what everyone else but you seems to have.

Even though issues relating to infertility have started to "come out of the closet" in recent years, the media has remained focused on primary infertility. This leaves women experiencing secondary infertility feeling alone, misunderstood, and subject to a variety of hurtful comments like "You should be grateful you have one child; some people have none," or "Your child is already four years old—don't you think it is time to have another one?"

What many people do not understand is that not having a second child is a very big loss for you. As each test comes back with less-than-good results and as each treatment fails, the loss of your second child becomes more real and more painful. Contrary to what some people might try to tell you, having one child cannot make up for the loss of the second child you want so desperately.

As Bob Deits explains in *Life after Loss,*

> Never apologize for grieving. . . . Learn to acknowledge that your loss is worthy of grief. Whatever your experience is, you must endure your very real feelings of sadness and anger on the way to recovering a full life once more. If you are going to come out of grief a better person, you cannot be concerned about how you ought to feel on the way through it.[3]

One of the best ways we know of to find understanding and acknowledgment for grief is to find others who feel just as you do. Through a secondary infertility support group, talking with other secondary infertility patients, or by working with a private therapist (specializing in infertility or loss) you can find people who will acknowledge your feelings and help you find the answers to the questions you confront everyday.

1. Should We Adopt?

We have been experiencing secondary infertility for about four years. My daughter is now seven years old and really set in her ways. In fact after all this time, we are all pretty set in our routines. Even though there is a lot of comfort in our nice orderly life, no matter how hard I try, I cannot help but feel like something is missing. I know I feel this way because I really want another baby. In fact I always thought I would have at least three kids. I come from a large family, six kids all told. I loved being around my brothers and sisters. Sometimes I think my siblings were even more important to me than my parents. So I want to give my daughter, my husband, and myself all the fun that I once had, a house filled with kids, toys, and commotion.

But I'm beginning to believe that the only way I can fulfill my dream is to adopt our second child (I am thirty-nine and hear the biological clock ticking louder than ever before). I feel very leery about adoption though, so I go back and forth, teetering between deciding on more medical treatments or contacting a lawyer and pursuing adoption. I'm afraid I would not be able to love an adopted child as much as my own. I also don't know anyone who has both a biological and an adopted child, but I would think the adopted child would always feel different and maybe like second-choice. I see too many problems. Can you tell me how other families have coped with this?

We can see that you are dealing with a lot of difficult issues all at once. Perhaps the best way to get to the answers you're looking for is to take each of your concerns and address them separately.

Almost everyone develops their concept of the ideal family as they are growing up. For some, like you, their vision will match their own childhood experiences, while for others the picture may be quite different. However, once a couple begins having children, things often change. Many couples are surprised to find discrepancies between what they thought would be the perfect family and what they are comfortable with now. This holds true for infertile as well as fertile families.

When considering what would be the perfect size for your family today, you will have to take into account many factors that never entered into your original plan. For instance, as you stated, you are all pretty set in your routines now. Think about what effect a new baby will have on your family, your life, and your lifestyle.

Then, if you do decide to continue with your plans for a second child, you will want to weigh the pros and cons of medical treatment and adoption. In doing so, it will be important for you to confront your general concerns, as well as your fears of not being able to love an adopted child as much as you love your biological daughter. For most couples experiencing secondary infertility this is the big question, and one of the toughest hurdles to overcome.

It is quite common for parents to believe that they will not love their second child as much as their first, regardless of whether their children are biological or adopted. But usually after the second child arrives most people find that the love they have for each of their children cannot be measured or compared. It is helpful for all parents who want more than one child to realize that they do not have to divide their emotions equally among their children as if they were cutting up a pie. The truth is that you can love each child as an individual, for who that child is and what he or she means to you. One child does not take you away from the other. You will find that the well you take your motherly love from is limitless.

Once you have considered all this, if you do decide that adopting a child is an option, contact a local adoptive parents group and talk to people who have both adopted and biological children. Read as many books as you can on adoption that include discussions of this issue. Remember that all adoptive parents must take that "leap of faith" trusting that their instincts to love, nurture, and parent any baby will in fact be stronger than biology.

2. I Feel So Alone

My son just turned four years old yesterday. His birthday party was great, all the kids had fun, and the parents seemed to enjoy themselves too. I, however, felt uneasy a lot of the time because at least three of the moms who came were pregnant. I couldn't bear to be around them, watching their big stomachs as they talked on and on about pregnancy. It was so intense for me that I had to leave the room a few times. I went into my bedroom, shut the door, and cried. I really want another baby. And I would give anything in the world to be in those women's shoes. I loved being pregnant with my first, and I imagine that I would feel the same way with my second. But I have not been given the chance. I have been trying to have another baby for three years and just recently went through an IVF cycle that failed. I've been feeling really bad lately. I can't even enjoy my son because all I think about is having another one. We go to the indoor playground, we go to other kid's homes, we play at home, and all I can concentrate on is myself and my feelings. I feel so guilty because when I tell anyone about how I feel, they tell me I should be happy for what I have and not try so hard to change things. Are they right?

Although those around you seem to be doing a good job of making you feel guilty about your feelings, it may help you to see that in spite of all you are going through, you are doing a terrific job of keeping up with your son's normal routines, birthday parties, play dates, and so forth. No one can tell you how many children you should have or should want to have. Your desire to "change things" and have a second child is up to you, not your friends or your family. Try to give yourself a break, and understand that experiencing "tunnel vision" during infertility is necessary as you work to resolve the crisis.

Therefore, your problem does not lie in the fact that what you are feeling is incorrect or abnormal but rather in the fact that you are not being understood by those around you. By not receiving supportive feedback or acknowledgment of your losses you are left alone to find your own way through painful feelings that can be both difficult and confusing. So, we urge you to look in another direction for guidance.

Think about it for a minute: wouldn't it be great to have someone there who understands, is willing to listen and make life with secondary infertility more bearable? Many infertility patients have found the support they needed through RESOLVE, a national volunteer organization for those experiencing infertility. In RESOLVE you will find women who share many of the same experiences and feelings as you. They will understand, better than anyone else, that wanting a second child does not mean you are ungrateful for the child you already have. Unlike those you have spoken to so far, women with secondary infertility will not tell you to stop trying so hard to change things. They will understand intimately your intense desire for another child.

RESOLVE offers general meetings, support groups, and even play groups for secondary infertility patients. If you don't do well in groups—and many of us do not—there are also member-to-member contact systems and referrals to professional therapists. RESOLVE services are designed to help infertile individuals work through their infertility and find their own answers.

3. Is One Child Enough?

My son is a great little guy. He does well in school and gets along with almost everyone he meets. We are truly enjoying him and feel very blessed that things are so good. It took us about two years to conceive him, so when he was about one and a half, I knew that if we wanted a second child, within a reasonable amount of time, we would have to start the craziness again. Well, that was about four years ago. We've gone the whole route—inseminations and two failed IVF cycles. To tell you the truth, I am getting pretty tired of it all. Even though it would be nice to have another child, I think I am about ready to throw in the towel and just count my blessings. I would really be fine with one and so would my husband. The only thing that is holding us back from ending our medical treatment is the idea that our son will not have the advantage of having a sister or brother to grow up with. You've probably heard all those stories about only children growing up self-centered and selfish. My parents believe it is true because my cousin was an only child, and all she ever thought about was herself. So, they warn me all the time that Jimmy will grow up to be like Stacy if we do not give him a sibling. How can I argue with them if I believe it too?

Simons reports in *Wanting Another Child* that, like you, many people believe

> "only children" are somehow at emotional risk, even though research has documented many positives that correspond to being a single child, such as high achievement, high self-esteem, and academic and occupational success. A study of only children has confirmed that . . . such stereotypes as the only child as "selfish, handicapped, anxious, not fun to be with, egotistical, [and] at a disadvantage when it comes to making his own way in a world" are "long on myth, short on actual research."[4]

While it may be true that your cousin only cared about herself, as you can see, such behavior is not necessarily a direct result of being an only child.

We have met only children who are wonderful company and very giving of themselves to others. Likewise, we have encountered many self-centered people who grew up in large families. How a child behaves is not determined solely by how many siblings he or she has. Children's behaviors are influenced by a wide variety of factors including basic personality, life experiences, and most importantly how he or she is being raised by his parents and those around him. For example, many families with one child make special efforts to reach out to other families with children, cousins, and so on to make sure their child has the opportunity to form close attachments that can mirror sibling relationships.

We need only to look at how you worded your question to see that your son is in no danger of following in the footsteps of your cousin. Your first two sentences say it all: "My son is a great little guy. He does well in school and gets along with almost everyone he meets." Since you expressed contentment with having one child, perhaps it is time for you to really listen to your own words and recognize that you and your husband are doing a wonderful job and that your son is turning out just fine, "even" without a sibling.

4. How Can I Get My Wife to Stop Obsessing?

My wife and I have a beautiful little girl. She means everything to me. My wife has wanted another baby for quite a while, but for some reason, still unknown to the doctors, we have been unable to conceive again. At first my wife seemed to accept the fact that we would have only one child. She was sad and disappointed, but she seemed to be handling it pretty well. Now, however, things have changed drastically. Having a baby is all she can think about. Her friends that are pregnant with their second or third child are driving her crazy, and she refuses to go to birthday parties if she knows another pregnant mother will be there. I tell her all the time that I do not want another baby, but she doesn't believe me. I really think she is getting irrational because our daughter is going to enter kindergarten this fall and she doesn't want to return to work. However, I have told her she doesn't have to, that we can afford for her to stay home and continue to take care of our daughter. I don't know what else to say to her. Maybe you can figure out how to stop this.

Though it may be difficult for you to witness your wife's intense emotions surrounding her infertility, it may help you to know that there is nothing unusual about her behavior. Her earlier reaction was quite mild considering that she desperately wants another child.

Like you, most men generally do not react as strongly as their wives do to secondary infertility. Many men feel content having one child, believing that the rewards as well as the responsibilities of one child are enough. These men have no problem creating their lives as a family of three.

Women often view secondary infertility quite differently. Your wife is the one who will not experience pregnancy again, and for most women this can be devastating. She is also the one who sits in play groups or at nursery school functions with other women able to get pregnant. Being surrounded by fertility is a constant reminder of what she cannot do and cannot have.

In addition to losing her dream of a family composed of more than one child, she may also be feeling guilty about not being able to produce a sibling for your daughter and another child for you. Even though you may have told her repeatedly that you do not care whether you have another child, given her situation, she simply cannot understand how that could be. Most women believe that such statements are said only to make them feel better and have nothing to do with the truth.

If all these reasons are not enough to get your wife upset about her infertility, consider this: on the first day of school, you will probably see your daughter off on the bus and resume your life as usual. Your wife, however, will not. Her day will be different than it has been for the past five years. She will return home to an empty house, knowing that kindergarten marks the beginning of the end of your daughter's total dependency on her. That kind of anticipatory loneliness can bring up intense thoughts and feelings about infertility. After all, your wife expected to be caring for another child by the time your daughter went to school. She never expected to be alone yet. Going to work may seem like a good idea to some people, but for women like your wife it is almost a punishment. It is "instead" of the child she wanted.

Your wife needs time to deal with her own loss, and she needs to do it in her own way. The best thing you can do for her right now is to support her by acknowledging her feelings. You can tell her that even though you do not really understand how she feels, she has a right to her pain and frustration. This will open the path to better communication between the two of you. By recognizing and supporting her grief process, as well as openly discussing the situation, you will most likely be helping her get to her own resolution quicker. You may also want to encourage her to join a support group or see a therapist or counselor to help her resolve her grief. Be patient with her and yourself.

5. What Should I Tell My Daughter about My Infertility?

My daughter is six years old and is in first grade. One of her assignments was to make a poster entitled "All About Me." We made this beautiful, colorful masterpiece filled with drawings and photographs of our vacations, her recitals, and her grandparents. The teacher liked it so much she hung it in the hallway. I thought my daughter would be ecstatic with all the praise she received from the teacher, but instead, she came home so upset, she could not stop crying. She explained that every other child in her class had put a picture of their brother or sister on their poster, and she realized that she was the only one in her class without a sibling. She wanted—rather demanded—to know why she could not be like the rest of the kids. I had no idea what to tell her. Do I tell her the truth, that I have been trying to have a baby for the past four years and have gone through four failed IVF cycles. Do I tell her how badly I want another baby, how much I would like to give her a sibling? You should probably know that we are still trying to conceive and will keep trying for as long as I can stand it.

Because your daughter's assignment caused her so much distress, we believe this would be an appropriate time to tell her about your mutual desire for another child. Given the age of your daughter we would be surprised if she was not already aware of your infertility on some level. According to Pat Johnston, author of *Taking Charge of Infertility*, "Secrets are almost universally impossible to keep. An undercurrent of whispers and overheard bits of conversation, of hesitant or evasive answers to questions, combine to drive children into a fantasy world which can be much more disturbing than reality!"[5] Parents who are not open about their infertility also run the risk of having their children believe that they "are deliberately depriving them of a brother or sister. They may even fantasize that they are at fault, that their 'bad' behavior has led to their parents' refusal to have more children."[6]

How much you want to tell your child will be up to you and your husband. Only the two of you can best judge what your daughter can understand and how she might react to your explanations. Since you have not mentioned anything to your daughter thus far, you may have some anxiety about doing so. Talking about conception is not easy for any parent, but talking about not being able to conceive can bring to the surface your deepest feelings about your infertility. Even if you are usually able to control your emotions, you may find it difficult to hold back your tears as you actually say the words you have held in for so long. If this happens, try to keep in mind what Simons wrote in *Wanting Another Child*: "Some parents project their own feelings of loss onto their children and fear that the children will share their distress and pain. Many children do express the desire for a sibling; while the words may echo your yearning, the emotional weight is not the same."[7]

Being open to answering your daughter's questions in simple and honest terms and bringing up the subject periodically at appropriate times will go a long way toward helping her deal with any effects the infertility will have on her.

3

Communicating
Effectively in Crisis
Gaining Understanding
and Support from Your Spouse

Seldom or never does a marriage develop into an individual relationship smoothly and without crisis. There is no birth of consciousness without pain.

—C. G. Jung[1]

*T*he setting: Mary, a thirty-something-year-old woman, sits on the couch thumbing through the newspaper with an impatient look on her face. She hears the front door opening, looks up, and sees her husband, Joe, hanging his coat in the closet.

MARY *(annoyed):* Oh, look what the wind finally swept in.

JOE *(equally annoyed):* Honey, I tried to reach you after I got the message that you called, but the answering machine wasn't on.

MARY: What time was that? I know it wasn't this afternoon because I called you right after I spoke to the doctor and then I waited around to hear from you.

JOE: I don't remember the exact time it was when I called. I was so busy all day, I didn't even eat lunch. Mr. Ross called me in for a meeting which ended up being a whole-day affair. He's driving me nuts. Now he tells me he is not satisfied with my department's progress and he wants me to figure out a way to increase their morale so we can increase sales.

MARY: Joe, do you even care what the doctor said, do you even give one flying——that I've been waiting all week to hear this news? All I ever hear about is your work.

JOE *(trailing behind her, enters the kitchen):* I'm sorry, honey. Really I am. What did the doctor say?

MARY *(annoyed, turns to look at him and stands with her hands on her hips):* He said what he always says, he said the test was negative. Don't you think I would have called you again if I had good news? I can't do this anymore. It's too much for me. Besides, nothing ever works for me, Joe. How nice it must be to sit at your desk and not think about me or about our infertility. You don't care about any of this, do you?

JOE: How many times do I have to tell you that I do care. I want a baby too. I just don't let it get to me. Look at you, you're a wreck. You never want to do anything except sit around and talk with your friends about how miserable your life is. How *horrible you have it because we don't have a baby. (His voice starts to grow louder.) Right now I have to concentrate on getting my career together. Stop this craziness. All I ever hear is negative things from you, day in and day out. Can't you see what it's doing to us?*

Mary, you will get pregnant, it's just a matter of time. Listen to what the doctor has been telling us. It could take a few tries. Give it some time, honey. Think more positively.

MARY: *And how do you propose I do that, Joe? How the hell can you expect me to think positively now? (She begins to cry.)*

Where are they going with this conversation? Will it escalate to the degree that neither Mary nor Joe has a clue about what the real issues are—the real hurt, pain, and grief?

Most couples probably believe that the reason they chose each other as life partners is because they thought alike and handled situations in a similar manner. While that might be true at the beginning or during the honeymoon stage of most relationships, feelings change as daily life begins to intervene. When a serious crisis like infertility hits, many couples find to their dismay that they are separate individuals with very separate styles of communication.

In the example above, Mary feels that her life is on hold right now. For her, infertility holds many meanings, most of which have a great impact on her self-esteem. She believes that having a baby will fix her life after years of feeling like a failure. She would like her husband to be as committed and have as much investment in parenthood as she does. However, for Joe, parenthood does not hold the same meaning, so he is able to focus on his work. Although he would like to be a parent, he believes his responsibility right now is to build a strong career so that his wife and his future children will be well provided for. (As we mentioned in Chapter 1, studies have shown that men begin to perceive infertility more like their wives do only after the third year of trying to conceive.)

To understand why men and women interpret infertility differently, we have to take a step back and see that men and women have a different style of communicating in general, no matter what the issue, no matter what the crisis.

According to Deborah Tannen, author of *You Just Don't Understand,* men engage the world

as an individual in a hierarchical social order in which he [is] either one-up or one-down. In this world, conversations are negotiations in which people try to achieve and maintain the upper hand if they can and protect themselves from others' attempts to put them down and push them around. Life is then a contest, a struggle to preserve independence and avoid failure."[2]

Women, on the other hand, approach the world where

conversations are negotiations for closeness in which people try to seek and give confirmation and support and to reach consensus. They try to protect themselves from others' attempts to push them away. Life, then, is a community, a struggle to preserve intimacy and avoid isolation.[3]

Of course, these are generalizations. Women obviously seek high positions and men seek connections, but men and women usually have different goals when communicating. Go back to the example of Mary and Joe to see what we mean. Mary's goal is to get Joe more connected to her. She desires his support and understanding. She needs to converse about her feelings regarding the failed cycle in order to sort her emotions through, not necessarily to find solutions to her problems. Joe's goal, however, is to protect and defend himself against Mary's accusations of not being a caring man. He tries to convince Mary that he is a good guy through his commitment to his job and by providing for her and their future family.

How did this happen? How is it that men and women view the same situation from such different angles? According to John Gray, in his book *Men Are from Mars, Women Are from Venus,* each gender comes from opposite places because we are supposed to; it is part of the plan, "the higher order." But many times we forget that we are predestined to be different, and we try, with all our might, to get our partners to be like us. We argue, resent, judge, and ridicule because the opposite gender does not think, act, or react in a similar fashion. The truth is we do not *instinctively* know how to support each other. This is why Joe does not understand why his attempts to help his partner fail. Many men are like Joe. They think that when a woman gets upset, they are being loving and supportive by making comments that minimize the importance of the problem. They may say (or imply, as Joe did in the above example), "Don't worry, it's not such a big deal." Or they may completely ignore the problem, assuming that they are giving the woman the "space" she needs to cool off. They don't understand that this kind of support makes women feel minimized and ignored. When women are upset, they want to be heard and understood.[4]

In the same scenario, it is also easy to see how Mary is misunderstanding Joe.

When Mary asked Joe to talk about the problem, she was assuming he would respond with empathy not advice. She felt angry, confused, and generally unsupported.

When you are angry at your spouse, upset about a situation, or in the middle of a crisis, it can be very difficult to communicate effectively, let alone supportively or lovingly. That is why we have included techniques on how to communicate better with your spouse that incorporate the differences between male and female styles. The questions below from couples specifically address the impact infertility has had on their marital relationship.

The Chinese define a crisis as a danger combined with an opportunity for change. If you as a couple are having trouble communicating during your infertility, you can take this time to see where the problems in communicating lie and find a way to fix them. Then you will know that in the future, you can make it through other life crises, no matter what they are.

1. My Spouse and I Have Different Perspectives

WIFE: My husband never wants to talk about our infertility and I try not to talk about it too much. But sometimes I need to discuss things with him and he just puts me off.

HUSBAND: My wife never stops talking about the infertility. It's one thing after another with her. The books, the doctors, the RESOLVE meetings. I'm sick of it, I don't want to hear it anymore. I've tried to tell her this, but she keeps going on and on.

This is a perfect example of how two people who most likely love each other deeply and who both want a child badly, perceive their infertility differently. According to Harville Hendrix in *Getting the Love You Want,* "although we all agree in principal that our partners have their own points of view and their own valid perceptions, at the emotional level we are reluctant to accept this simple truth."[5] Instead, we try to make our spouse wrong, believe that our own way of thinking is right, that there is no other way. Aaron T. Beck, M.D., in his book *Love Is Never Enough,* agrees:

> Sometimes partners work themselves into such opposing positions that they
> seem incapable of reaching even a compromise. They dig their heels in, sticking
> stubbornly to their own point of view. They see their own views as eminently
> reasonable and those of their partner as unreasonable. Above all, they cannot rec-

ognize or acknowledge that their partner's wishes or complaints might be sig-nificant.[6]

So, how can a husband and wife who take opposite sides of an issue come to a middle ground where both parties can feel acknowledged despite the crisis they find themselves in? Below is a role-reversal exercise. Its purpose is to help you imag-ine what it would feel like to be in your spouse's place and walk in his or her shoes. We have listed situations common to both women and men experiencing infertil-ity. Read them over and ask your spouse to do the same. Then take some time to think about each situation before discussing them.

FOR THE HUSBAND[7]

- If your wife finds out she did not get pregnant this month, see if you can un-derstand how she feels by imagining that:

When you were a young boy, you wanted to be on a team, you worked out for weeks, practiced with family and friends, ate the right foods, took vitamins, and so forth, and the day of the tryouts you did your best—in fact you thought you did great—but sadly you did not make the team.

- When your wife cries all night long that her sister got pregnant, see if you can understand how she feels by imagining:

When you were a teenager, all your friends had cars, and you badly wanted one also, but you just did not have enough money to buy it. So you asked your parents and grandparents for money, and even asked your sisters and brothers to contribute to your savings. One day when you came home from school, you saw a new, used car in your driveway. Convinced your parents had fulfilled your dream, you ran into the house cheering, screaming, jumping up and down that you finally could be like all the others. But you stopped dead in your tracks when you learned that your parents did not buy it for you, but gave it to your brother instead. They told you they felt you were just not ready yet.

- When your wife gets so anxious waiting for the results of a pregnancy test that she cannot focus on anything else, see if you can understand how she feels by imagining:

You felt pretty confident after you interviewed for your very first job. Everything went so well that you could hardly believe it. You wanted this job. It would offer you everything you dreamed of, everything you had worked so hard to prepare for. They told you they liked you and you had a good chance of getting it. But of course, they had to interview others, and would let you know their final decision within a week or so. You sat by the phone every day hoping they would call and let you know so you could move on with your life.

- When your wife is pregnant for six weeks and then has a miscarriage, see if you can understand how she feels by imagining:

You got the job of your dreams and everything was going along well: you finally had money in your pocket, so you bought yourself a car, rented an apartment, and even booked a vacation. One morning you walked into work happy and content, and your boss called you into his office. You figured it was about the promotion you expected to get, but instead he told you the company was not happy with your performance. He fired you on the spot with no warning.

Now for the Wife

- When your husband tells you he is angry because you do not listen to his suggestions for how to solve your infertility problem, see if you can understand how he feels by imagining:

When your best friend has a problem, she calls you every day to tell you how badly she feels, how her world has been destroyed. But each time you say something to help her see it from another perspective, she says you are wrong. You try to rephrase your suggestions so she can understand you, but she insists you still don't know what you are talking about.

- When your husband says he is angry because no other problems besides the infertility seem important anymore, not even his problems, see if you can understand how he feels by imagining:

A friend of yours has a serious problem with a relationship. She had been dating her boyfriend for five years and they seemed really caring and loving of one another. She had told you many times that they would eventually be married, but then something happened and the relationship ended. And now she talks about it incessantly. No matter what the situation is, or the conversation is about, she always brings the subject back to her problem.

She makes you feel as if your problems pale in comparison to hers. They are not even worth talking about. It is as if you don't exist.

• When your husband tells you that getting pregnant is not the most important thing in the world, that you should move on and look at other ways to create a family, see if you can understand how he feels by imagining:

Your sister calls for the fourth time today—the seventeenth time this week—to tell you about the same problem she has had forever. Her boyfriend is mean to her, never calls when he is supposed to, never gets her presents or takes her out. But for some reason, she will not break up with him. You encourage her to move on, telling her there are other fish in the sea. But she tells you she loves him and that she would do anything to get him to change. She knows it sounds stupid, but that is how she feels.

By switching roles, even momentarily you might be able to understand the frustration, loneliness, and disappointment your spouse is feeling. A whole new world can open up to you. As Hendrix says, "Marriage gives you the opportunity to be continually schooled in your own reality and in the reality of another person."[8]

2. All She Ever Does Is Talk about Our Infertility

I have proof now that my wife is obsessed with our infertility. All she wants to do is talk about it day and night. She calls me at work to talk about it, she calls her mother, her sister—anyone and everyone who will listen. I really need a break. We had been planning to go to Hawaii for years, and finally we have enough money. But she won't hear of it. She wants to do another IVF cycle instead. I want coconuts for my money, not needles. Any suggestions?

Like many spouses you have expressed a need to take a break, a vacation from the daily routines of life and from your infertility. Unfortunately this request has fallen on deaf ears because in your wife's mind there is no down time, no time to let go and have fun, especially no time to take a vacation. A vacation could mean a missed cycle, a missed opportunity.

What your wife is experiencing, however, is not uncommon. Like infertility, where stress levels are equal to that of cancer and AIDS, many patients feel obsessed or at the very least preoccupied with the pursuit of resolution. They have to. It is what helps them to stay focused on getting through the rigors of the medical treatment. Since your wife seems desperate to talk about the infertility, give her what she needs rather than fighting her. Make time for her whenever possible. We know this might be difficult for you but we believe that this is a temporary situation due to the crisis of infertility.

With regard to your desire for a vacation, you might want to plan a trip that can be more spontaneous than a Hawaiian holiday. For instance, go for one that can taken with very little planning between the time a treatment is completed and the time you are expecting an answer.

3. He Just Doesn't Seem to Hear Me

It happened again today. I asked my husband last week to come with me to my doctor's appointment and he said he would. Then this morning, I mention that the appointment is this afternoon and he says he can't come because he has a meeting. He swears I never told him, but I know I did. To be honest, it's not just appointments. I don't think he listens to anything having to do with our infertility. It's getting so frustrating. I don't know what to do anymore.

It's difficult to feel like you are not being listened to when you are conversing about a subject as important to you as infertility. Most of us take listening for granted. We do it so often and so routinely that we assume that we do it well, especially around those we love. However, good listening is a skill that needs to be developed. Therefore it might be useful for you to ask your husband what you could do to help him remember appointments. Does he need you to write him a note, call his secretary, or leave a message on his voice mail a few days before the appointment? It might also be useful for you and your husband to learn a technique known as *mirroring,* which helps couples to send and receive clear and simple messages to each other. Specifically, it helps to counteract the speaker's feelings of being unheard by training listeners to listen more carefully. We have found that couples who have implemented this technique into their conversations have clearer and more effective communication.

Here are the directions for mirroring, taken from Hendrix's *Getting the Love You Want.*[9] The brackets show where we have altered the examples to fit the needs of the questioner.

1. Choose one person as sender. Have that person say a simple statement that begins with the word "I" and describes a thought or feeling. For example, "I woke up this morning and felt anxious about going to [the doctor]."
2. If the sentence appears too complex, the "receiver" can ask for simplification: "Could you say that in fewer words?" Once a clear and simple sentence has been sent, the receiver paraphrases the message and asks for clarification. Example: "This morning you woke up feeling that you [didn't

want to deal with another treatment, another consultation at the doctor's office]. Did I understand what you said and [how you were feeling]?" (Asking for clarification is important, because it shows a willingness to try to understand.)

3. The sender responds by saying, "Yes, you did," or by making a clarifying statement such as "Not exactly. I woke up this morning wanting to go to [the doctor's, but only if I would hear good news]." This process continues until the sender acknowledges that what was said and thought and felt has been accurately communicated. (This exercise will feel like an unnatural, cumbersome way of relating, but it is a good way to assure accurate communication.)

4. Switch roles and communicate another simple statement. Practice this technique several times until you become familiar with the procedure.

4. It's No Fun Anymore

My wife and I used to do so many things together: parties, walking on the beach, shopping, even bowling. But those places are filled with children, so just going makes us feel terrible. Is this how it is going to be until we resolve our infertility— no fun, no life?

Like you, most people who experience infertility for a prolonged period of time begin to limit their fun to child-free activities. This is understandable since seeing children and families is a constant reminder of what you do not have but so desperately want. However, it sounds like putting these limits on your activities has created another loss for you. If this is true—if not having fun and spontaneity is compounding your sadness—it might be time for you to find new ways to enjoy yourself. Hendrix, who is a renowned marriage therapist, says that having fun can fortify your emotional bond to one another and deepen your feelings of safety and pleasure. And while you are experiencing a crisis like infertility, feeling closer to one another can surely ease some of the pain. The following "fun list" exercise is a way to help you do this.

Begin by making separate lists of fun and exciting activities you would enjoy doing as a couple. Include face-to-face experiences and the kinds of body contact that may be physically pleasurable such as tennis, bicycling, dancing, taking a walk, and so forth. Share your lists and make a third list combining all your suggestions. Pick at least one activity to do each week.[10]

Obviously the activities you both chose will be the easier to do, but make sure you try each other's suggestions for new and different activities. Even if you or your partner feel a bit reluctant to let go and have fun, see if you can push each other to try new things. Taking a break from infertility, even for only a few hours a week, is important for both your emotional and physical health.

5. There's Conflict in Every Part of Our Lives Now

My husband and I have a bit of a stormy relationship, but we've always been able to work things through on our own. Lately, however, we've been fighting a lot. At first it was mostly about infertility, but now it has spread into every area of our lives. What we buy, who we socialize with—everything seems fair game lately and it's beginning to worry me. I don't know if it's the infertility or if we are really heading for a divorce. I just can't tell anymore.

What you are experiencing must be very scary for you. We know how complicated infertility makes your lives and that fighting during this crisis can be downright unsettling—unless you can begin to view what is happening as an opportunity for you and your husband to learn new ways of interacting and loving each other.

According to Nancy Van Pelt, author of *How to Talk So Your Mate Will Listen*, "learning how to fight fair might be the most important communication skill you will ever learn."[11] Try to stick to the subject at hand. Do not allow yourselves to drift into other issues, especially those you dig up from the past. If at all possible, stay away from name calling, put-downs of appearance or intelligence, and interrupting. Obviously there is no room for physical violence in conflict resolution.

While discussing the problem employ the mirroring techniques described in question 3. Once the problem has been defined and feelings have been aired honestly and openly, you can start the conflict resolution phase.

1. Begin by discussing all the possible solutions.
2. Next evaluate the options and narrow your alternatives to one, two, or three possible solutions.
3. Choose the best path, which usually requires compromise from both partners. Pay attention to make sure that one partner is not the full-time compromiser. This process is not about winning and losing, but rather about finding a solution that feels right to both of you.
4. Implement the solution you have agreed upon by writing down the specifics of the agreement. For instance, if you have decided to take a break from infertility concerns and go away for a weekend, write down whose responsibil-

ity it will be to make the travel arrangements, who will pack, who will take the dog to the vet, and so on.

While discussing the problem and trying to integrate the techniques mentioned above, one or both of you might experience anger, frustration, and confusion. These feelings can be so strong that you might want to run away from the pain by leaving the room. See if you can hang in there; don't walk away yet. Most likely, if you can last for just a few minutes more and can stick to the ground-rules, your resolution will come.[12]

If you find that you cannot reach a common ground, we suggest you seek out a marriage counselor. Having a third party present helps many couples to resolve their differences.

4

Family and Friends
Living in a Fertile World

You pick up the phone and hear your college roommate's voice on the other end. The panic begins immediately when she says the words you have avoided hearing for weeks, "Hi, what's new? Did you get the test results yet?"

In your attempt to answer her question you feel yourself stumbling over your words and shutting down your feelings so you won't let on how badly you feel that yet another cycle hasn't worked. Why is this happening? you wonder. How could such a simple, well-intended loving greeting send you spinning into an anxiety-ridden state? Could it be because she has two children and you believe she would not understand? It never used to be like this . . .

Infertility changes you. It is a time when you find yourself disconnecting from those you love the most, your family and friends. A time when you pull back from the world and focus inward because isolating yourself can actually feel better than remaining a part of the fertile world.

It is not as if you want to separate from those around you; in fact, you want to be right in there with them, a part of the fertility club that includes your mother, your sister, friends, even the next-door neighbor's fifteen-year-old daughter. But you have no choice. The gap between you and the fertile world widens, and it becomes harder to be around those who now seem to disappoint you at every turn with their inaccurate medical advice, offhand remarks, and insensitive responses to your grief. Their comments, all well intended, serve to increase your already intense feelings of anger, disappointment, sadness, and especially envy.

Even the most sensitive people you know probably won't understand what you are going through. Because fertile people only know about infertility from news and talk shows, which present the condition from a medical viewpoint. When they make uninformed comments—telling you things will be all right if you just see the right doctor and find the right treatment—they don't realize they are adding fuel to your already raging fire.

And whenever they reignite your fire with their questions or unrequested input at family functions, on the phone, or even in the hallway at your office, you may feel as if you want to disappear. You beg them, silently, not to bring up the dreaded subject, because if they do and you have to respond, all those horrible feelings of being inadequate and different will rear their ugly heads. In defense you temporarily pull the plug on your relationships, leaving you separate and apart. This disconnecting of relationships is like an old-fashioned switchboard with all the wires unplugged and left hanging. All the energy that used to run through those wires, all the passion must now go toward combatting your infertility.

Some people disconnect physically. They don't go to baby showers or christenings, and turn down any invitations that might involve "family talk." Others disconnect by performing a brilliant emotional disappearing act, becoming numb inside so the pain will not hurt as badly or deeply. (Refer back to Chapter 1 for a more detailed discussion of this.) One woman told us:

> Even though we had been trying for two years, the doctors kept telling me I would get pregnant soon. My sister believed them and because she wanted us to have our children together she went ahead and started trying to get pregnant. And of course she did the first month. After that, I didn't want to see her or even call her. No matter what she said, it was never right; it always felt hurtful or just plain wrong. Even when she would say she was sorry that we didn't become pregnant together, I didn't see her disappointment. I just felt like I hadn't lived up to her expectations. I remember crying to my husband, hysterically, saying, "How could she do this to me? She should have known to wait until I was pregnant." That was five years and two children ago. Sometimes when I look back at that time, I can't believe how bad I made her out to be. I wanted her to put her life on hold all those years just because mine was, and that wasn't fair or realistic. But at the time, I was hurting so bad I just couldn't help it.

Infertility patients develop very sensitive antennae regarding relationships. They can often spot a hurtful comment coming even before the other person starts to speak. Some infertility patients keep score cards in their heads, tallying up who around them is the most perceptive and insightful, and who says the most hurtful remarks.

But as difficult as it may be for you to deal with the fertile world, your infertility can also become a no-win situation for your family and friends. The people around you, like the woman's sister quoted above, may want to be sensitive and supportive to your needs, but may be unable to. As one infertility patient told us, "When asked what my family and friends can do for me, I tell them, 'just *ask me how I am*,' and when asked what my family and friends should not say to me, I tell them, '*don't ask me how I am*.' "

It can be equally difficult for fertile people to share their lives with you right now. Often friends and family will be aware that their pregnancies and children are making you uncomfortable even if they do not understand exactly why you feel that way. They may also have difficulty witnessing the pain and grief you are experiencing and may find that your crisis is bringing them dangerously close to feelings that are too uncomfortable for them to handle. So they avoid you or at least avoid talking about the subject of your infertility. Instead, they do what they know best—offer quick-fix solutions to your problem or anecdotal accounts of their friends' daughters' successful pregnancies from fertility drugs. Such comments leave most infertility patients feeling misunderstood and alone and only serve to push you farther away from them. And because it is very rare for either side, fertile or infertile, to verbalize their feelings about each other, the disconnecting often becomes a two-way street, paved with misunderstandings.

And what becomes of these friendships and family ties strained so much during your infertility? Luckily we have found that most of the time the people you moved away from will "stay on the line" and wait for your return after the crisis of infertility is over. It is an amazing phenomenon which we have seen happen over and over again. With the arrival of resolution there comes a peace to relationships that at one time seemed damaged beyond repair.

It may help you to get through this time of working toward resolution, if you can remember two things: (1) "all our relationships are hedged with ambivalence—we love and we envy; we love and we compete";[1] and (2) no matter how much family and friends might want to help or how much they try, they cannot take our pain away, even a little. Expecting them to is asking the impossible. Therefore, like most infertility patients, you may need to look to others for the acknowledgment and support you need. As mentioned earlier, one of the best ways to do this is to join a support group.

There has been mounting evidence that group support, and social support in general, can lead to an overall healthier view of life and sometimes can even save lives. One ten-year study, led by Drs. David Spiegel and Irving Yalom at Stanford University, proved such findings. The doctors led a support group for women in treatment for metastatic breast cancer. Their goal was to help the patients cope with the overwhelming nature of living with a fatal diagnosis. After one year, the doctors found that the women attending the group experienced less emotional trauma than other female patients who did not participate in a support group. However, the most remarkable results occurred ten years later. After contacting the women who participated in the group, Spiegel found that they lived an average of twice as long as the control group.[2]

This is obviously very impressive, exciting news, and you will be happy to know that we have observed many important benefits from participating in an infertility support group. Walking into a support group or a general informational meeting for the first time is not easy, but hearing other people say *exactly* the same things you say, feeling *exactly* the same way you feel, and experiencing the *exact* same reactions from their family and friends as you is like seeking shelter in the eye of the storm. These meetings become a place where you can let your guard down and feel comfortable to express those emotions that have had to go underground in the "fertile world." As one woman said,

> Going to my first RESOLVE meeting was so wonderful. Even though everyone there had different kinds of medical problems, our emotions were the same. I finally felt like I belonged somewhere. It had been so long since I had that feeling.

At these meetings you will almost always find at least one person you can relate to, and most people find many more. (You can find the address and phone number of RESOLVE in Appendix II). RESOLVE's belief that "You are not alone" really summarizes their goal of helping others find not only emotional comfort but medical and insurance information as well. RESOLVE also recognizes that not everyone is comfortable in groups. If this is true for you, the organization will refer you to a therapist specializing in reproductive loss and individual therapy.

It is important for you to remember that, for now, you are in the midst of a crisis, and one of the most helpful ways you can navigate this wild course is to find others in the same boat. It may be hard to take that initial step because it requires admitting that you are part of a group you did not choose to be a member of. However, once you reach out, you will find that, as psychotherapist and grief specialist David Treadwell implies in his lectures, *grieving alone hurts much worse than grieving together.*[3] Find those people who will help you get through the process, and when you do, you will clear your path to loving and accepting your family and friends, even during this most difficult time.

1. How Can I Survive My Sister's Baby Shower?

My sister and I have always been very close, even though she's five years younger than me. I can remember even as children we would talk about living on the same block, getting pregnant at the same time, and raising our children together. Now we do live on the same block, but she's pregnant and I'm not, and I don't know if I ever will be. We have been trying for over four years now, and nothing seems to be working. My sister's pregnancy has been very difficult for me, it's hard even to look at her as she gets bigger and bigger. It's not that I don't want her to have her baby or that I don't wish her the best. It's just that we were supposed to do this together. As her only sister, I am planning to give her a baby shower. But honestly I don't know how I am going to get through that day. Is there anything I can possibly do to make the day easier for me?

In light of everything you are going through, hosting a shower for your sister is very commendable. However, the fact that you are a loving sister does not mean that your feelings are to be ignored and pushed aside. Like you, most people who are infertile try to feel happy for someone who is pregnant while struggling with their own feelings of jealously and sadness at being left behind. This internal struggle creates anger—anger at oneself for feeling bitter and envious, and anger at the situation infertility has put them in.

In order to keep your relationship with your sister free of misunderstandings and unnecessary hurts during this difficult time, we suggest you talk with her about your feelings and your sense of loss. Be as honest as possible about her shower and what it means to you. Since she has lost a dream as well, she will probably be very understanding and may even share much of the hurt you are feeling.

If after talking with your sister, you decide that giving her a shower would be too difficult, you might want to ask a close relative or friend to host the event. On the other hand, if you believe that you are capable of giving her the shower, there are a few pointers we can offer you:

- As hostess of the event, you have the advantage of being in control, so consider delegating those responsibilities that would be most uncomfortable for you. Asking someone else to shop for the decorations or to write out the invitations may be just what you need to get through the planning stages of the shower.
- To make the day a little easier you may want to invite an ally to the party. A supportive friend can help you get through those dreaded yet inevitable childbirth and labor conversations.
- If a conversation does become too difficult, your hostess status will allow you to leave with the excuse that you need to attend to some aspect of the party such as the food or drinks.
- Bringing a video camera to the baby shower is another great way to distance yourself from the group. Staying behind the camera gives you something to do and allows you to move about the room freely without being obliged to listen to any conversations that may be difficult to hear.
- It is tradition in some families for the sister or the woman who "gives" the shower to help the guest of honor open the presents. For many infertile women, this is the most difficult part of the shower experience. If this is true in your

family, it is time to break the tradition. Plan ahead and pass the honor on to your mother, close friend, or relative. If you think your sister will notice, be sure to talk to her about it before the shower.

No matter what you decide or how you plan the day, there will be times when it will be difficult to be there and times when things will go very well.

2. They Never Told Me about My Cousin's Pregnancy

My cousin has been pregnant for the last eight months, and no one bothered to tell me because of my infertility. They said they didn't want to make me feel any worse than I already do. I can't believe they kept this secret for so long, I am absolutely furious. The only reason they finally told me was because the baby shower invitations were in the mail!

There is nothing worse than feeling isolated from your family, the people you depend on for support and understanding. Your family sounds as if they withheld the information about your cousin's pregnancy in order to protect you from more pain and sadness. Perhaps they have always been overprotective of you as you were growing up. If this is the case, they will most likely continue to do so whenever a crisis situation arises.

Therefore, you need to decide how you would like to be treated in the future. Ask yourself if you would feel better knowing about a pregnancy as soon as everyone else knows. If so, who would you want to hear the news from (your mom, your sister, or the pregnant woman), and how would you want to be told (over the phone, in person, or through an invitation to the baby shower)?

Once you have decided which scenario feels best, talk to your family and let them know how you want things handled in the future and how important this is to you. Although they might not agree with you at first, eventually they will feel better knowing exactly what you need and want rather than trying to second-guess what they believe would be best for you.

3. My Infertile Friends Are Becoming Parents

After years of dealing with our infertility on our own, I finally decided to join a women's infertility support group and honestly, it was the best thing I've ever done for myself. The friends I have made through the group and the support they have given me has meant so much to me. No one else, not even family, comes close to understanding my feelings the way these women do. My problem, however, is that my two closest friends from that group are about to become parents, one through a pregnancy and the other through adoption. I am feeling terrible, I know I should be happy for them, but I'm not. I got very used to having them to talk to about all my infertility, and now I will be back to having no one.

The impending changes in your friends' lives are bringing up those old familiar, painful feelings of loss and envy. Therefore it is important for you to decide whether you can deal with this situation, since no matter how hard you try to push the feelings away, they will remain a part of this relationship until you find your own resolution.

Before you make that decision, however, consider that you are assuming your friends no longer want to discuss infertility with you. And this may not be true. Remember that the intense feelings of infertility don't vanish the moment you decide to adopt or get a positive pregnancy test. (See Chapter 11.) In fact, you may be surprised to learn that even women who have completed their families, through adoption and/or the birth of biological children, report that infertility remains an issue for them. (See the Epilogue for further discussion of this issue.)

Since the three of you have probably shared many personal insights in the past, it would not seem unreasonable to be honest about your feelings now. One group of friends from a RESOLVE support group had such a discussion and agreed that the woman continuing medical treatment would be the one to decide when and if to have contact. If she was having a particularly difficult time in treatment, such as right after a failed IVF cycle, she could decline an invitation to see her support group friends. However, if she was feeling hopeful and having an easier time with her infertility, she could choose to socialize with them and give what she could to the friendships.

If you decide, however, that you cannot deal with the prospects of these two friends becoming mothers at the same time, you need to know that you are not alone. Many women find it too uncomfortable to remain friends under these circumstances. Some people in a support group build friendships based solely on their infertility and have little else in common. Therefore, when one person gets pregnant or adopts a child, the relationship can lose its common ground.

If this is the case, you might want to join another support group or attend lectures that deal with the medical and emotional issues of infertility. Since you have been able to cultivate support from these women, there is nothing prohibiting you from meeting another group and doing the same again. At this point in your life, you need to do whatever is best for you to get you through the crisis.

4. My Relatives Say Such Rude Things!

My husband and I have been trying to conceive a child for over four years now—even IVF hasn't worked for us. Recently we were at a family reunion, and the subject of our childless status came up, as it does at every family gathering. This time, however, some of our cousins made some really rude comments, basically implying that we don't know how to "do it." We were shocked, and so hurt we couldn't even speak. I wanted to leave the picnic immediately. It was hard enough seeing all my pregnant cousins and the babies in the first place, but this made things ten times worse. My husband was able to calm me down and we stayed for another hour, but the whole time I couldn't wait to leave. It was a nightmare.

Like you, we have found that uncaring, rude, and hurtful comments are an inevitable part of the infertility experience. We don't know of anyone who has missed being offended at a social occasion or a family function. Although such encounters are painful, finding a suitable way to deal with them can make all the difference in the world for you. By "suitable" we mean finding ways to approach the situation with some sense of control.

Merle Bombardieri, in her book *The Baby Decision,* talks about "The Victims' Bill of Rights." You may want to apply these to similar situations that are bound to come up. At all times you have the right:[4]

- To choose whether or not to discuss your situation with a particular person.
- To be heard if you do wish to explain yourself to chosen people.
- To cut the conversation short or change its direction.
- To point out and object to the techniques a pushy person is using on you.

If you do decide to tell the person about your infertility, you might start by letting him or her know how much you want children and that you are doing everything possible to conceive and/or adopt a child. If this does not help, the person most likely is not listening to you and you can refuse to talk further, knowing you did your best. If you decide not to discuss your situation with this person, it might help to have a rehearsed comeback so you will always have something appropriate to say. Some people choose to use humor in this situation; others prefer to change the direction of the conversation by putting the questioner on the defensive. For example, if someone asks if you are ever going to have children, you might say, "What is it about my not having children that bothers you?" Although we cannot predict how every person will respond, this tactic should cause most people to think twice before making inappropriate comments in the future.[5]

Remember, you have the absolute right to decide how you want to handle conversations about your infertility. It is a very personal matter and should be treated accordingly.

5. They All Say Relax and I'll Get Pregnant

How do you respond to people who say, "Relax and you'll get pregnant"? Are these people serious? I have been trying to get pregnant for over six years. Do they really think I haven't been relaxed even once during the seventy-five or so cycles we have been trying? Does this make any sense?

This is probably the most common advice couples receive from those "trying to help." Saying "just relax" minimizes the seriousness of the problem and implies that you, not your medical condition, have caused your infertility. These kinds of quick-fix, offhand remarks are difficult to hear and bring up angry feelings for all of us who know better. You can, if you wish, deal with that anger by letting people know you are willing to do everything within your power to resolve your problem including stress management, but that their belittling of the problem is not helpful. You can also tell them that, although stress and infertility can be related and infertility does cause stress, it is still not clear what role, if any, stress plays in causing infertility. As research continues to show that stress reduction has a positive effect on pregnancy rates, infertility patients are increasingly employing these techniques as an adjunct to their regular medical treatments, not as a substitute for them. Stress reduction may not only increase their chance of getting pregnant but also have a positive effect on their general health. People who have tried methods such as meditation, visualization, or simple breathing exercises report feeling calmer and more able to handle the intense commitment infertility makes on the couple and individual. (See Appendix I for a description of these methods.)

By approaching negative comments in this way, you may finally be able to put them to rest. In the meantime we urge you to take full advantage of any course of treatment that might at best increase your chances of pregnancy and at the very least help to ease the stress during this very difficult time in your life.

6. They Say Adopt and I'll Get Pregnant

Three months ago my wife and I decided to end medical treatment and pursue adoption. Since that time, I can't tell you how many people have told me my wife will get pregnant as soon as we adopt. Although it seems highly unlikely that this will happen to us, people insist that it will. Everyone seems to know someone who this has happened to. Whenever they say this, I don't know what to think, what message they are trying to send me. Are they trying to tell us not to adopt, to wait a while longer? Or are they telling us to do it, so that we can get the biological child we had originally tried to have? Don't they understand, we no longer care where our children come from? What should I say to these people?

If you are finding that these comments are making you angry, it is probably because this statement usually contains the underlying message that adoption is second-best to pregnancy. It is true that most adoptive parents who experienced infertility desperately wanted to be pregnant and have a biological child. But as time went on, they realized that being a parent, having a child in their lives to nurture and love, was more important. Most adoptive parents tell us with all their heart that the baby who came to them was fated to be theirs—that all the years of turmoil were well worth the wait for *this* baby.

It is also a common misconception that adopting a child means you will finally achieve a pregnancy. Pregnancy after adoption occurs in about 5 percent of all cases. And even in those situations, pregnancy most likely would have occurred with or without a prior adoption. Obviously, if you and your wife were fortunate enough to become pregnant after you adopted, you would be doubly blessed.

If you find yourself in this situation again, there are a number of things you can say. The first is to educate these people with the statistics previously mentioned. The second is to explain to the person that enjoying parenthood and loving your child will have little to do with giving birth. The third option is that, instead of answering their question, you can make a joke, change the subject, or choose to disengage.

7. They Blame My Wife's Infertility on Her Career

My wife has been getting very little support for our infertility simply because she is a lawyer. Many of our friends and family seem to have the attitude that, because she initially chose her career over motherhood, she is now "paying the price" for waiting too long. Though my wife is hurt by these comments, she continues to believe that they are right. I have tried to tell her they are wrong, but so far she seems to be on their side. Is there a better way I could deal with these comments so my wife wouldn't believe them so quickly?

Your wife is lucky to have a husband as caring and concerned as you. Like you, many men want to be able to protect their wives from painful comments. Although we know this comes from a very loving place within you, the reality is that infertility hurts—even if you were able to stop all the horrible comments, your wife's pain would still be present.

Help your wife to see that these kinds of harsh remarks are quite often rooted in jealousy and tell more about the person saying them than the person receiving them. It may be hard to fathom how anyone could be jealous of your situation, but remember that your ability to work on your careers, travel freely, and take advantage of whatever money and time afford you can be upsetting to those who cannot make a move without a child following behind needing physical, emotional, and financial care. Even though these people would never really give up what they have, to them your life may seem very attractive.

Your might also share with your wife the fact that her infertility is not a political issue. She does not have to stand in the line of fire for those who wish to prove that motherhood should come before career.

Like most infertile women, your wife would no doubt benefit from having her feelings validated. Talking to her about what her life might be like today if she hadn't made the choices she made may be the first step in a long process of acceptance. You might ask her what she thinks it would feel like to be infertile *and* have no career, or how it would feel to not be able to afford the advanced medical treatments so often not covered by traditional insurance plans.

You also may be able to find the support you both deserve through participation in a support group. (See our list of groups in Appendix II, the Resource Guide.) There your wife will most likely find many women who choose to have their careers first. The self-exploration the support group affords will help both of you come to terms with your feelings about infertility. Then, whenever the insensitive comments come your way, you can put them in their place.

8. Do I Have to Go to the Baby Shower?

I have been trying to get pregnant for three years now, and I am not dealing with it very well. When I got an invitation to my cousin's baby shower, I thought it would be too difficult to go, so I decided not to. When I told my mother I wasn't going, she got angry and said my cousin would be very disappointed. (Translation: my mother would be very disappointed.) Then she said, "You know, you can't hide forever." Now I honestly don't know what to do. I know my mother is right, but I'm afraid I will end up crying through the whole thing.

You are dealing with two issues: your mother's disappointment at your not going to the shower, and your feelings about "hiding" from the fertile world because of your infertility.

Let's deal with your mother's feelings first. For one reason or another, your mother would feel let down by you if you did not attend the baby shower. Although there could be a number of underlying reasons why this might be the case, in our experience some mothers feel obliged to follow family protocol, which in your case means cousins are expected to attend their relatives' showers no matter what. Your mother realizes that if you are not at the shower, she will be the one put on the spot. She will have to decide how much or how little to share with your relatives about your situation.

This is where you might be helpful. If you decide not to go, let her know what you want her to say. Do you want her to tell them about your infertility, or would you rather she tell them you are ill? Think about it and advise your mom accordingly.

The other issue your mother mentioned, which seemed to hit a nerve with you, is the problem of isolating yourself from the fertile world. This need to remove yourself from potentially painful situations is extremely common and normal for people experiencing infertility—or any crisis situation. Why would anyone want to stick their hand in a burning fire?

One way to get through this feeling of wanting to run away from painful situations is to think about how to best take care of yourself. First, validate your feelings and understand that you actually do have a choice in the matter. If you decide to attend the shower, figure out the best ways to get through the day. If you decide not to attend, comfort yourself with the fact that you are doing what is best for you now.

One woman used a visualization exercise to help her decide whether or not she should attend a shower. She imagined watching the pregnant woman open her presents in front of all the guests. Because this literally made her sick to her stomach, she knew the present opening would be the most difficult part. She decided to attend the shower anyway, but left early, before the gift opening. Another person, who did the same exercise, realized that the talk about babies and labor would be intolerable. She opted not to go to the shower and decided to spend the day at home with her husband.

What are you anticipating to be the most difficult part of the day? Play the scene over in your mind as if you are watching a TV show. Then, like the women mentioned above, try to figure out a way to counteract the harsh effects. Through visualization you may see that you are able to handle attending.

If you are really not ready to tackle such a challenge, try not to feel too guilty—most women experiencing infertility do not go to all their family functions.

Whatever your choice, there is no need to punish yourself for making the decision to take care of *you*.

9. Why Won't My Mother Talk about DES (Diethylstilbestrol)?

Because of my infertility problems, my doctor suspected I might be a DES daughter. Even though my mother never remembered taking DES, I was lucky enough to find the records, which confirmed that she had in fact been given the drug. When I told her, she changed the subject, and every time I've mentioned it since then, she does the same thing. I told her I don't blame her—after all, how could she have known what the doctors didn't even know? Until now we've never had trouble talking about anything, she was always so open and honest with me. Why she is acting this way?

It is great that you are not blaming your mother for taking DES while she was pregnant with you. However, she is probably feeling responsible for your problem. Your mother, like the other 4.8 million women who took DES, did not know at the time that the drug they were taking to prevent miscarriage would have such far-reaching consequences. Unfortunately, many of these women still feel guilty, even though it would have taken a psychic's wisdom to have known the drug would cause many of their children to experience miscarriage, premature labor, ectopic pregnancies, and infertility. As one woman said, "The doctor was God . . . you always did what you were told."[6] To complicate matters further, your mother is probably feeling resentment toward doctors and fertility drugs. She may believe you are falling victim to the very same system that promoted DES thirty years ago. You can imagine how helpless she must be feeling.

To offer your mother support, give her and yourself some time to sort out her emotions. You might find that you, too, are angry and resentful that your mother put you at risk, even though you know rationally that she was not aware of the effects. It may be helpful for you and your mother to air these feelings. In time, the anger and resentment will dissipate.

In the meantime, you might want to get yourself some support and information from DES Action U.S.A. and your local RESOLVE chapter (listed in Appendix II). There you will meet other DES daughters and may even be able to arrange for your mother to speak with some of their mothers.

10. My Sister Calls Me Self-Centered

My sister is no longer speaking to me and my husband. She has decided we are self-centered because we couldn't bring ourselves to attend her son's first birthday party. At the time, we were undergoing our fourth IVF cycle and were not hopeful that things would go our way. In the past we have always attended every holiday gathering, but we felt like we just couldn't do it anymore. I have tried to explain to her how we feel, but she says she's tired of listening to me complain. I am so hurt, I don't want to lose my sister, but why can't she see my side of this?

Both you and your sister have the best of intensions at heart; an invitation to a child's birthday party and a decision to avoid a painful situation. So why did you both get so hurt? It could be that both of you forgot to understand each other. Do you understand why it was so important for her that you attend her son's birthday? Does your sister understand why it was so important for you to stay away? Perhaps the best way for the two of you to resolve this is to work toward understanding each other.

Tell her how you feel. Let her know that not attending her son's birthday had nothing to do with her or your feelings about your nephew, but rather was an attempt to avoid painful feelings that you are not able to cope with now. The key word is "now" since this situation is temporary. Tell her you look forward to the days when you can go to her home for her son's birthday with an open heart and mind.

Let her explain to you how much her son's birthday party meant to her—why your being there was so important and how sad she is that she cannot celebrate such an important day with her sister. She may even tell you she feels guilty that she has a precious child while you are still struggling to conceive.

Sharing these thoughts will enable the two of you to put this incident behind you and come to some agreement about how to deal with similar problems, which are bound to arise in the future.

If the two of you cannot come to an understanding, then it might be time for you and your sister to look at the history of your relationship. Are there other unresolved feelings you two have never talked about and resolved? Being brave enough to put deep-seated feelings on the table for examination can lead to a deepening of your relationship.

11. I'm Feeling Left Out

Ever since my younger sister became pregnant, she and my mother spend hours comparing notes on their pregnancies. Who had morning sickness, who craved what foods, and on and on. I've tried to change the subject, but my sister keeps going right back to pregnancy talk. I used to be so close to my mother, but now all I feel is anger when I'm around her. Don't they see me sitting there without anything to say?

It is extremely difficult to cope with a pregnant sister or sister-in-law, especially when the sibling is younger than you. To some degree we all maintain our birth-order roles even as adults. Older siblings are usually expected to lead the way by being the first to attend college, get a job, get married, and have children. This explains why your sister's out-of-birth-order pregnancy may feel like it has threatened your place in the family. Especially your place with your mother, who has not yet found a way to balance her joy over your sister's pregnancy with your need to have the pain caused by your infertility acknowledged.

According to Gay Becker, in *Healing the Infertile Family,* "Relationships with mother and daughters are complicated at the best of times. But a woman's experience is different from her mother's when she is having no success with conception. This difference may potentially strain communication. Yet this is a time in her life when a woman wants to feel especially close to her mother. A woman needs her mother now. For many reasons."[7] Right now you need your mother to be there for you too. Have you let her know how isolated you are feeling? Your mother cannot read your mind; she needs *you* to tell her. Let her know what it is like for you to sit with her and listen to all her pregnancy stories without having anything to contribute. Even if she does not understand infertility and all the feelings associated with it, she may still be able to give you the support you need.

If your mother cannot be a source of support, all hope is not lost. Support groups and therapists that specialize in loss and infertility cannot replace your family, but they can help you cope better with feelings of isolation.

12. All My Friends Are Passing Me By

Kathy, Mary, Renee, and I have been friends since elementary school. We've gone through everything together. Seven years ago I was the first one in the group to get married. Four years ago I was the first in the group to announce we had tossed our birth control out the window and were going to start our family. Today my husband and I have temperature charts, tests, treatments, and drugs but no baby. My friends, on the other hand, are all married. Kathy has one child, Mary has two, and Renee just called to tell me she's pregnant. Now I know all our conversations are going to be about pregnancy and babies. We are all supposed to get together for dinner on Saturday, but I am seriously considering not going. I feel like my infertility has taken away everything, including my friends.

Sharing with your friends the pain and frustration you are feeling may seem risky, but doing so may in fact help you to judge what role they can play in your life during this difficult time. As Robert Veninga says in his book *A Gift of Hope,* "Some will not understand what you are going through. Others will not care to know. And still others will be more interested in telling you what to do than in listening to your problems."[8] You will know right away which friends understand your pain. Those who listen with a sensitive ear and ask you questions out of concern and not judgment will probably be there for you in ways that others cannot. However, the key to maintaining friendships is the recognition that a lack of understanding is not necessarily grounds for dissolution. Your friendship may remain highly valued for its history. Friendships based on shared history are important because they keep our roots steady during the torrents of infertility.[9]

To take the pressure off yourself and this group of friends, consider cultivating other avenues of support specifically for your infertility. The kind of relationships that develop in a support group are "cross-roads friends,"[10] whom you will be able to share your feelings and stories with. They will understand the rigors of testing, the ups and downs of treatment, and what it feels like to be disconnected from your family and friends.

You may be lucky enough to develop intimate, long-term friendships with some of these people. Such friendships can only arise from revealing your private self. Infertility, like grief, lends itself to this sort of relationship because your feelings may be closer to the surface than they have ever been before. And if you feel comfortable enough, this is a good opportunity for you to share feelings that have been difficult and painful, such as jealousy, envy, and being different and alone.

Your question reveals that you have been blessed with good friendships in the past. We hope you are brave enough in the future to get the support you need.

13. Going to Family Gatherings Is Getting Too Difficult

During the first four years of our infertility my wife and I attended every holiday celebration our families planned. Although we never hosted these events, for fear that we wouldn't be able to make a quick getaway, we were usually able to stay for most of the festivities. After each event, we both felt incredibly drained, and my wife usually cried the whole way home. All that talk about babies and kids, watching them open presents on Mother's and Father's Day, and even ringing in the New Year while my sister-in-law nursed her newborn baby has been rough on both of us, but especially my wife. While we love our families, these obligations are getting harder to manage. I'm trying to convince my wife that maybe we should go away during Christmas this year, but she says it wouldn't be the same. The same as the horrible times we have had for the last four years? How can I convince her that going away may be the answer we have been looking for.

Although your idea of getting away for the holidays is a good one and one we recommend to many people in the midst of infertility, your wife does not see it as a viable option right now. Your wife's family, like most others, may believe that holidays should be spent together regardless of individual circumstances. For your wife to ignore such a rule, may make her feel she has in some way betrayed her family. Therefore even though it may be difficult for you to see her suffer through another holiday, hold on to the idea that she is not saying no to the vacation because she doesn't want to please you; rather, she is unable to be "disloyal" to her family.

Knowing this may help you find other ways to cope with the holidays. Below is a list of strategies we have compiled from a variety of resources. You can employ these or work on creating some of your own.

1. Try to socialize with other child-free couples during the holiday season.
2. When you go to holiday gatherings, arrive after the children have opened their presents. You will avoid watching all the hoopla over the children and might even have the opportunity for an adult conversation.
3. Celebrate the holidays in your own home first. Get a tree, light the menorah, and so forth. Give each other special gifts—after all, you are going through a very difficult time and need to celebrate your love for one another.

4. Volunteer your time during the holidays. It can take your mind off your pain for a little while and will give you the feeling that you have done something worthwhile. Decide on a charity you both feel strongly about.

5. Rehearse comebacks for dreaded questions. For instance, if you know that your Aunt Nancy will inevitably question you about your not having any children, come up with a response beforehand. Also, plan some strategies that will get you out of situations that seem intolerable. For instance, one couple we knew used their beeper whenever they wanted to leave a party. The wife would find an unoccupied room with a phone and page her husband. He would answer the call and inform the hosts that they had to leave because of an emergency.

Remember the holidays are for *you* too. Stay in touch with how many things you have to be grateful for: family, jobs, health, and most importantly each other. Do the holidays your way.

14. How Can We Find a Balance between Privacy and Secrecy?

My wife and I have been trying to have a child for the past three years. So far we have told no one what we are going through. I am scheduled to undergo surgery for a varicocele next month, which will require me to take some time off from work. We feel like we will now be forced to tell a few people, but we are not happy about it. Do you think I should lie to people about the nature of my upcoming surgery?

How much you allow others to know about your infertility is up to you as a couple. Some people feel that infertility is an intensely personal issue and may have very practical reasons for feeling this way. For instance, some couples need time to come to terms with their infertility before telling anyone else. Others want the freedom to make decisions regarding their treatment without opinions or interference. Still others may be undergoing treatments that violate their families' religious beliefs.

Some couples choose to keep their infertility from others because they are embarrassed and ashamed of their situation. They believe they have failed to meet others' expectations. They hide physically and/or emotionally and pretend there is nothing wrong when in fact they are experiencing the biggest crisis of their lives. When these are the motivations for secrecy, remember that you've done nothing wrong; you did not cause your infertility.

Before you decide to share any information regarding your infertility, you and your husband should explore exactly why this secrecy has been, and continues to be, so critical. If your reasons are practical, you may want to continue as you have been. However, if you are running away from your reality because of negative feelings about yourselves, it may be helpful to openly discuss how infertility has affected each of you. (See Chapter 1 for a discussion on infertility and identity.)

5

Working 9 to 5
Balancing Career and Baby Making

In writing this chapter, we remembered how, during our own experience with infertility, our jobs had become a veritable minefield of painful comments and reminders of our struggle. At the same time our careers also offered us a much-needed respite from thinking about how much we wanted a baby. Such conflicting sentiments about work shared by so many infertility patients are reflected in the questions throughout this chapter.

While work may seem like one of the last places to be affected by infertility, it is in fact one of the first. That first appointment with an infertility specialist signals the beginning of a delicate balancing act in which time must be made for both work and infertility. As couples progress through testing and treatment, they may find it harder to concentrate on work, and colleagues may notice their distracted behavior and frequent absences from the office.

Infertility patients must decide early on what, if anything, to tell co-workers, how much time off is reasonable to ask for, how to maintain quality relationships with fellow employees and employers (especially pregnant ones), and how to attend office baby showers and company family picnics without visibly falling apart. Infertility patients must become proficient actors to get through the times that require putting on a happy face.

Infertility also causes many patients to rethink their careers. They may find it necessary to pass up a promotion if the added responsibilities will limit their treatment choices and make them less available for procedures like inseminations or IVF. Furthermore, occupational hazards that might cause infertility and miscarriages, such as unhealthy chemicals, gases, or equipment, have led some people to quit or alter their jobs to limit their exposure. At the same time, infertility patients can also find themselves unable to leave a job they dislike because they need their insurance coverage during this period of intense medical treatment.

Some jobs are just so emotionally incompatible with infertility that facing work each day becomes an incredible challenge. The career responsibilities of obstetrical and pediatric doctors and nurses, teachers, child-care providers, and teenage pregnancy counselors are just some of the professions that demand tremendous emotional stamina from the infertility patient. In addition, those who work in management positions must be able to put their personal feelings aside when dealing with matters concerning families or pregnant employees.

Many women also report that they left or wanted to leave their jobs as the demands and stresses of infertility multiplied. Women in very high stress careers or in jobs that did not offer enough time flexibility to undergo treatment sometimes changed careers or rearranged their jobs into part-time or job-sharing positions. Some found it necessary to take a leave of absence.

As difficult as these issues seem, there is hope. In this chapter we show how you can begin to manage your work environment so that it stops managing you. One way to do this is to find a balance between thoughts and feelings, and *reframe* those situations that give you the most trouble. By challenging your negative thoughts throughout the day you will be able to deal more effectively with the world around you.

For example, many people we have spoken with report that when something at work reminds them of their infertility, such as a pregnant co-worker talking about her baby shower, their whole day or possibly even the whole week is ruined. By reframing the situation, patients can look at such conversations in this way:

> *A typical work day is eight hours. The conversations about babies or pregnancy took at the most five minutes. Am I willing to allow a five-minute conversation ruin the other seven hours and fifty-five minutes?*

Of course, the vast majority of people experiencing infertility would be upset for a while. Depending on where you are in your medical treatment, this unsettled feeling can last a long time. The key is to literally throw yourself back into your work as quickly as possible; diverting your attention from infertility to what is right in front of you at the moment is vital. Tell yourself that your work is very important—not necessarily more important than your feelings, but nevertheless meaningful. You can and should deal with the anger, jealousy, and any of the other normal emotions that might arise at work—when you get home that night. At that point you can write about the experience in a journal or share what happened with a spouse or friend, which will be more productive than dealing with these intense emotions at work.

Finally, it is important not to define yourself by your struggle for parenthood or forget what your job originally meant to you. Remember that infertility is not a career but a time-limited crisis. Work can give you a sense of accomplishment, restore a sense of purpose during a troubled time, offer financial security, and even allow you to get away from your struggle with infertility, even if only for a little while.

1. Should I Stay at This Job for the Benefits?

I had it all planned. After graduating from high school I was going to work for a little while, then get married, buy a house, have children, and quit my job. I always wanted to be a stay-at-home mom. Almost everything worked out. I got a job as a secretary after high school, then got married. We saved enough money to buy a house and then tried to get pregnant. Now three years later I'm still trying to get pregnant and I am stuck in a job I hate because we need the money and the insurance coverage to pay for all my infertility treatments. I wake up every morning upset because I don't want to go to work. What should I do?

It is clear that in the past you have been thoughtful, persistent, and hard-working. These are the same skills you will need to continue to get through your infertility.

Just as you planned all the things you needed to do before you started your family, it is now time to plan the steps to take to resolve your infertility. Having a "plan toward resolution" will enable you to feel more in control of your life, and give you the information you will need to manage your career until your infertility is over. Your Plan toward Resolution may have many steps, or it may be as simple as: "I will go through three more IVF cycles and then start looking into adoption."

In addition to deciding what steps your plan will include, you will want to estimate out how long your plan will take. Then you will be better able to figure out if you are willing to stay in your job for that long. The issue of medical coverage may keep you in your present position for a while longer than you want to, but knowing when you can quit your job should make it much more bearable.

In the meantime, keep busy by updating your resume, talking to employment agencies, and following the want ads. You might even want to consider taking some courses to brush up old skills, add new ones, or start preparing for a new career.

2. Thoughts of Infertility Get in the Way at Work

I have become so obsessed with my infertility that I can't stop thinking about it. Even in the middle of my work, I find my thoughts drifting to my problem, and sometimes I begin to cry. It's so embarrassing some days I just want to quit.

Like you, many infertile women find themselves crying at inopportune times, and describe their preoccupation with infertility as obsessive. The inability to concentrate that you describe has led some infertility patients to quit their jobs. Although the majority of women continue to work, the fact is that just about everyone has difficulty handling the combined stresses of work and infertility.

Although there are times throughout the day when you can't concentrate, there are probably many more times that you can. Thinking about your work or socializing with your co-workers gives you the opportunity to get away from the stress of your infertility. In addition, your work may help you maintain your self-esteem at a time when your infertility may threaten it.

If there are good reasons to stay at your job, you need to figure out how to manage and take advantage of your workday. The following techniques may help you deal with some of the situations you face at work.

KEEPING ORGANIZED: DAILY INFERTILITY LISTS

The first thing you might try is to get up a few minutes early each day to make a list of all the things you need to do concerning your infertility. Then write down when you think you can accomplish each item. Try to limit their intrusion into your life to periods before work, during lunch, or after work. This way you won't have to keep remembering to do things throughout the day.

INFERTILITY JOURNAL

The second thing you may want to do is to start a daily *infertility journal,* in which you write how you feel about your infertility. You might also want to look ahead and imagine what might cause trouble for you, such as a pregnant co-worker, a baby shower at the office, or calling about test results. Write down your truest feelings, and include ideas for coping with these situations. This will give you the resources and the strength to get through the day.

EXERCISE

Lunch hours do not have to be spent engaged in conversation. Going for even a short walk after lunch can relieve some of your pent-up stress and give you time to be alone with your thoughts.

FOCUSING EXERCISE

You may want to use a focusing exercise whenever you feel your thoughts drifting. By thinking about where you are right now and everything you are doing at the that moment, you will be able to get your thoughts back on track quickly (see Chapter 1).

Anytime you find yourself crying during the day, remove yourself from the situation, either by going to the ladies room or by closing your office door, to give yourself a few minutes to calm down and get yourself together again. Recognize that you are going through a very difficult time and that some days are going to be harder than others. It is important to be good to yourself.

3. How Do I Cope with a Pregnant Employee?

I've been trying to get pregnant for the past five years during which time I have worked my way up to supervisor at an agency that employs twenty-five people. Until recently I was able to keep my feelings about infertility out of the office. Then the other day my assistant informed me she was three months pregnant. I was so upset, I even thought about firing her so I wouldn't have to look at her everyday. How am I going to get through the next six months?

Since this is the first time your feelings about infertility have surfaced in the office, it would be meaningful for you to look at both the timing of the announcement and the person involved. Think about what is going on in your life right now that was not happening the last time someone announced a pregnancy. Are you scheduled to undergo a test or treatment that might be painful or difficult? Have you been stuck in one stage of your infertility and feel hopeless or confused? These are the kinds of situations that may be contributing to your anxiety over your assistant's announcement.

Also to be considered is your relationship with her. Perhaps you are beginning to perceive her as more successful than you, even though your position in the office should tell you otherwise. In a way, this is similar to the younger sister getting pregnant while the older sister struggles with her infertility (see Chapter 4). Both can be very disorienting because they seem to defy the natural order of things. Keep in mind that feelings, positive and negative, are usually stronger toward those we are closest to than those we are care less about. Like those living nearest to the epicenter of an earthquake, your proximity to this person may be causing greater upheaval than those at a distance experience.

To help you cope with your fears about the future, you may want to begin by taking stock in yourself again—who you are, what your strengths are, and what you are all about. Ask yourself if it is really true that you cannot make it through this pregnancy. Recognize how much you have already been through, and tell yourself that you will not allow this one issue to stop you dead in your tracks. Certainly you will need all your strength to do this and to keep it up for months, and some days may be more difficult than others. However, you did not get to your position without an ample reserve of strength.

We also recommend talking to your assistant. Begin by being open and honest, saying something like, "I'm happy for you, but this is really hard for me." Tell her what you are going through and your feelings about it. Even though some people prefer to keep silent about their infertility in the work environment, in some instances honesty works best. It can open the door to two-way communication and an easing of pent-up feelings.

By looking at the reasons behind your anger and discomfort with your assistant's pregnancy and by working toward a more open relationship, we believe you will be better prepared to handle the next six months.

4. Do I Have to Go to Office Baby Showers?

I have worked for the federal government for the last four years. Because my department is very large and employs mostly women, it seems like there is a baby shower every other week. While I don't mind contributing money for food and a gift, I really hate going to these showers. I don't want to listen to all that talk about labor, delivery, nursing, and diapers—it just depresses me more than I already am. I feel so stuck. If I don't go, they might think I don't like the woman or that I'm being a snob. What can I do?

You are certainly not alone in your dislike of baby showers. Most infertility patients hate these gatherings no matter who they are for. Every story about childbirth is a painful reminder of what they don't have right now. However, it may help to understand how useful a baby shower can be to the woman who is expecting. Most women are pretty good at hiding it, but the truth is that pregnancy is very scary, especially the first time. Will the delivery be difficult? Will I have a cesarean section? Will the baby be healthy? And will I be a good mother? These are just some of the many questions pregnant women face. While those going through infertility may ease their fears by joining a support organization, those going through pregnancy must look to others who have been there for guidance and support. By sharing their stories during a baby shower, other women tell the guest of honor that everything will be all right for her, just as it was for them.

Now you may be thinking, "Okay, I understand why women want showers, but I still hate them. What can I do about it?" From a practical standpoint, coming late and leaving early, or feigning work-related excuses, cuts down on the actual time you will have to be there. If you have any friends in the office, you might want to tell them how difficult these showers are for you and ask them to talk to you during the function about other things besides babies. If there is no one you can confide in, you may want to position yourself next to the single women without children or the men in the department in the hopes that even if the conversation does turn to babies, it will soon turn to something else.

Another tactic that you might want to try is to reframe the situation. Instead of looking at the baby shower as a horrible, difficult, and painful event, turn it into a call for action. One woman said after attending a christening, "After it was over and I had finished getting angry and feeling sorry for myself, I finally realized that it didn't really matter how fair or unfair it was. The only thing that mattered was that I wanted what they had, and I would do whatever I needed to do to get it. The next day I scheduled the surgery I had been putting off."

5. How Can I Deal with Insensitive Co-Workers?

I made the mistake of telling some people at work that I'm having an infertility problem. Now I'm being hounded with advice and jokes about how to get my wife pregnant. One guy said he could show me how to "do it right." I don't know how to put an end to these stupid comments.

It is unfortunate that the friends you confided in told other people about your personal life. At this point there is no way to stop your news from spreading, so the problem you now face is, what if anything you should say when your colleagues make these comments.

First realize that there is a difference between people who make jokes and insults and those that offer advice. The latter are doing so probably because they care about you. Even if the advice minimizes the seriousness of your problem or is outdated or superstitious, recognize the fact that they are trying to help and thank them for their concern. There is no need to go into elaborate explanations or detailed medical histories. By giving these people the benefit of the doubt you may find their comments easier to listen to.

As for those people who make rude comments about infertility, they need not be acknowledged. If the comments persist, you can rehearse some comebacks when you are calm so that you will not be caught off-guard.

6. A New Job . . . a New City . . . a New Doctor?

Yesterday my boss told me that the agency wants me to oversee their new of-fices in a neighboring state. All I said to him was "thank you" and left. I was too upset to talk. I knew that if I did take this position, I'd have to find a new doctor and would probably be too busy to get to the appointments. I never even thought about what a great opportunity this would be for me until I got home that night and told my husband. I am very confused.

Even though this would normally be a time to celebrate, it is understandable that you would be upset about all the unknowns that come with this promotion. In-fertility has a way of making us see only the negative side of things. Even positive occurrences can feel overwhelming in the tumultuous wake of infertility.

The trusting relationship you have built with your doctor is important, and you may feel it will never be duplicated. It is not surprising, then, that you are hav-ing a hard time believing that changing things could work out. But can they?

To help you make an educated guess about the possible outcome of your de-cision, make a list of all the negative and positive aspects, both personal and pro-fessional, about this job offer. You may even want to ask your husband or friend to help you with the list. Be especially sure that you are not using your infertility to avoid a formidable career move. Most importantly, don't be afraid to challenge the negatives. For example, your fear of having to switch doctors can be challenged by being open to the possibility of finding an even better doctor, with more flexible hours. By shining the light on all your fears you will be on your way to making the best possible choice.

7. Will Quitting a High-Stress Job Allow Me to Get Pregnant?

I have been trying to get pregnant for the past two years and am currently undergoing treatment. My job is very high pressured and I'm always feeling anxious there. Some days I don't know if I can handle the pressures of both the infertility and the job. Many people have told me that I would be able to get pregnant if I quit. I assume this is another way of saying "relax and you'll get preg-nant," so I don't bother to talk to them about it. Is there any truth to what they are saying?

No one knows exactly what role stress plays in causing infertility. Research has been slow in coming. Although there is a definite mind-body connection between certain conditions and illnesses, there is no scientific evidence that would support a decision to quit your job in order to get pregnant.

We do suggest you work toward eliminating as much stress as possible from your life since reducing stress is always better for general health. This does not necessarily mean you should quit your job though, since unemployment could prove much more stressful than working. Instead, evaluate your current position by asking yourself whether you are constantly feeling pressured, unhappy, or unable to undergo infertility treatments. If this is the case, then you have good cause to consider changing your current position.

Some women have told us that they felt much better after they left a stressful position and found a less demanding job. (Sometimes this meant going to a part-time job.) Their new jobs enabled them to accomplish their infertility treatment goals in a timely, less stressful manner.

Of those women who quit their jobs altogether, the ones who were happiest with their decision were the ones who had found ways to fill their days and sought outlets for their energy. Some volunteered, others spent time with their families, still others went back to school. The key, they found, was to find meaningful activities that kept them away from constant thoughts of infertility.

If you feel it would be better for you to stay at your job, think about ways to reduce your stress. While it may not get you pregnant, stress reduction can help you to feel more in control of your body and leave you less susceptible to other illnesses and conditions that might limit your life. The stress reduction techniques in Appendix I should help you not only during your infertility experience, but for the rest of your life.

8. Work Is Getting in the Way of My Doctor's Appointments

I work in a day-care center and it is very difficult for me to get time off. All of the infertility doctors in my area work the same hours as me, making it virtually impossible for me to see them. I only seem to have two alternatives, either I quit my job or I don't get pregnant.

Your situation is difficult but not impossible. Consider the following suggestions:

1. Check with your doctor for extra early appointments or Saturday hours.
2. Talk to your boss about getting someone to cover your classroom so you can take a long lunch break.

3. Consider going to a physician affiliated with an IVF program. These programs often have extended hours to meet the more intense demands of high-tech treatment.
4. A group practice, rather than a single practitioner, may offer you more flexible hours.
5. Be sure you have a complete list of specialists in your area.

If these things do not work, consider teaching a higher grade or taking an administrative position that will allow you a more flexible schedule. Working in a related field, taking a leave of absence, job sharing, going back to school, and taking a part-time job are also options to explore. Whatever you decide, your goal should be to maintain as much of a "normal" life as possible while undergoing treatment. Aside from the insurance benefits and financial income, most people report that work provides a much needed boost to their self-esteem and a diversion from the crisis of infertility.

9. I Have Trouble Relating to Fertile Employees

My wife and I have been undergoing infertility treatment for three years now. I find it hard to relate to my employees with growing families. Their constant family interruptions and child-care problems are very annoying and counterproductive. To make matters worse, three women will be on maternity leave within the next four months. Whether you are fertile or infertile shouldn't make any difference in job performance, but I am beginning to think it really does.

In trying to keep an office running smoothly, every manager runs into challenges. You have the added burden of trying to put your personal problems aside so you can work effectively with those who have children. In order to do this, you will have to learn to separate the external problems from those annoyances brought on by your personal frustration and anger about your infertility. Policies and their enforcement cannot be set up to discriminate against those with children. Most progressive companies are becoming more family-friendly by offering family leave time, on-site day care, and even job sharing.

On one level, the dilemma your employees face is similar to yours. As an infertility patient, you and your wife have had to take time out of your life and probably your work to undergo testing, treatment, and possibly even surgeries. Although your desire for a family has nothing to do with your desire to do a good job, these two things may make conflicting demands on your time. Likewise, it is not that your employees don't want to do a good job, it is just that sometimes they need time to take care of their families. Recognizing that the problems with your employees are actually time conflicts should help you look for practical solutions.

10. Get Me Away from This Pregnant Co-Worker!

One of my co-workers is pregnant again after experiencing two miscarriages. She talks nonstop about her pregnancy even though she knows about my infertility problem. She tells me what she's eating, what vitamins she's taking, how she has to rest—on and on and on. How can she be so insensitive to my feelings? If she was a friend I would just avoid her, but she is a co-worker, so I can't get away from her. What should I do?

Sometimes understanding people's feelings better helps in understanding why they say the things they do. For women who have had multiple miscarriages, getting pregnant is truly only half the battle. They often feel as infertile as women who have never been pregnant because there is no baby to take home. Indeed, the medical definition of infertility includes the inability not only to conceive a child but also to carry a child to live birth.

Like many women who have miscarried, this co-worker may feel she did something wrong during her last two pregnancies. To compensate for her guilt she is probably trying to exert as much control as possible by making positive changes to her lifestyle and diet. Most likely she is terrified of losing a third baby and may be receiving very little support for her apprehensions. Therefore, she may feel comfortable sharing this information with you because she knows that you understand her fears and share her passion for the precious nature of a pregnancy. While it might be difficult to socialize with her day after day, try to remember that you both share the same goal: to bring home a healthy baby.

11. My Boss Thinks I Have an Incurable Disease

My boss thinks I have an incurable disease because I'm always leaving early for medical tests and treatments. I want to tell him the real reason, but I am afraid he will write me off for career advancement if he thinks I am going to get pregnant and leave. Should I tell him?

This seems to be one of the most common and troublesome dilemmas working women face when undergoing medical treatment for infertility. Look at all your options before deciding whether to reveal the situation to your boss. Telling your boss about your infertility may lead him to believe that your only priority is to have a baby and leave your job. However, if you have been in his employ for any length of time and have proven yourself to be a valuable asset, he may think otherwise. It is up to you to convey your commitment to your work. If he understands that you intend to continue being a devoted employee, he might be more sensitive than you think.

In our experience, telling someone you trust who is in a position of authority will ease your strain and allow you more flexibility. Such people usually are willing to make allowances if you too are willing to compromise. This might mean coming in early, working late, bringing work home, or working on weekends.

If you decide you cannot reveal the true situation to anyone, you could simply say you are undergoing medical testing for something innocuous like allergies or back pain, or you can leave it open as unexplained symptoms.

12. My Job Exposes Me to Many Fertile Women

I am a pediatrician experiencing infertility, and I see pregnant women and mothers all day long. Usually I am able to keep my feelings at bay until I get home. The only time I have trouble in the office is when I see women who don't appreciate their pregnancies. I get so angry and distracted I find it hard to concentrate. I love my work and have a lot invested in my career, but I don't know how much longer I can stand it. What should I do?

People experiencing infertility often report having intense reactions to those who take pregnancy and children for granted. They describe feeling angry and confused about what to say or do when a negative comment is made.

First, do not expect yourself to leave all your feelings at home. Women experiencing infertility, especially those who work with pregnant women, cannot go for long without thinking about some aspect of their problem. Give yourself permission to feel the anger or resentment when people make hurtful comments. Then use the reframing technique suggested at the beginning of this chapter.

Second, find at least one co-worker who can support you during the difficult times when you need to talk. You may even be able to find others who are experiencing infertility problems.

As a physician, part of your job is to educate people. If it seems appropriate at the time, you could talk to the women making negative statements about their pregnancies to find out why they feel this way. You may be able to find help for those women who would benefit from counseling. The result would be job satisfaction for you and help for a mother and her child.

6

Dealing with the
Medical Community

*The Challenges of
the Infertility Patient*[1]

I walked into my first RESOLVE meeting with really no knowledge of infertility. I was getting pregnant—I certainly didn't believe I was infertile. I only had a postcoital test at my gynecologist's office: it wasn't exactly what you would call an infertility workup or anything. I just couldn't bring myself to make an appointment with a specialist. I kept saying one more month, next month. RESOLVE was a way of putting things off, or at least I thought it was. I was doing my research thing. Avoiding the experience in favor of collecting information. I was told it was a good way to learn about infertility.

That first night at the meeting, a specialist from one of the local hospitals was there. He talked about infertility and treatments and then fielded questions from the audience. Most of the questions were about the drugs and their side effects. One woman asked if infertility drugs would make hair grow on her face. I almost died. It was all downhill from there. I cried all the way home in the car. I didn't want hair on my face, I didn't want to take drugs, I didn't want to have this problem, I didn't want to be like "them." And in the forty minutes it took to get home I successfully convinced myself I wasn't like "them." I didn't look like any of them, they were older or something—anything—just not me. I continued to put off treatment for a while and didn't go back to another RESOLVE meeting for over a year. I found the meetings to be helpful and the information invaluable. When I needed to take Pergonal shots, my doctor never told me to numb the area with ice first. I found that out at a RESOLVE meeting. I took a lot of Pergonal shots that year; it saved me a lot of pain.

Eventually I learned so much at the meetings I got involved in the organization as a phone counselor. Two years later my husband and I did an interview for a local TV station doing a special report on infertility. That day I said to him, "Remember when I didn't want to even admit I was part of that group?" And he said, "Yeah, and now you're their poster child."

The process of accepting one's infertility is never easy. Like this woman, most infertility patients go through a period of denial when medical intervention seems too overwhelming—even entertaining the thoughts can set off the deepest of fears. But as time passes and the need for a child becomes greater, infertile individuals begin to see that opening the door to treatment also means opening the door to hope and possibilities. For many infertility patients, medical treatment provides the miracle they have always dreamed of.

However, moving through the world of reproductive medicine can be an arduous journey of painful tests and expensive treatments. It is a world fraught with many more questions than answers. Infertility treatment is as draining emotionally as it is physically. We live in a brave new world of options and hope but also many unknowns. The greatest of these is what effects these treatments and drugs will have in the long term, on us and on the children we produce. Conflicting research continues to be published in newspapers, consumer reports, and medical journals in this country and around the world. Thus it is up to patients to decide whether the unknown risks are worth taking for a pregnancy, which is why all couples considering treatment should become educated consumers.

Increasingly we have found more patients questioning the use of infertility drugs, demanding fewer cycles, and looking toward healthier alternatives. Couples today often move toward the higher-tech treatments such as IVF at a much faster rate than in the past, thus reducing the number of drug cycles and hopefully limiting any of the risks that may exist. We are also seeing a greater interest in stress management and alternative medicines as an adjunct to medical treatment.

This chapter discusses these trends as well as ways to help you get the facts and support your need to make informed choices. Take this information as a starting point for further research. The challenges of medical treatment are many, and no one book or even one doctor can provide all the insights and knowledge you will need to make your decisions. It will be up to you to determine your needs, explore your options, and find your own direction. Opening the door to information can mean opening the door to your dreams.

A NOTE ABOUT INSURANCE PLANS

Insurance plans and coverages vary tremendously from company to company and from state to state. We recommend that if you have concerns regarding insurance coverage, you get involved with the politics in your state by contacting your state legislators and by working with your local RESOLVE chapter. Many chapters have set up insurance committees to lobby for positive infertility and adoption legislation. On a national level, RESOLVE has also been lobbying for reform in these areas.

1. When and How Should I Choose a Specialist?

I am thirty-five years old and have been trying to get pregnant for three years now. My gynecologist has taken a few tests and found nothing wrong. She put me on Clomid hoping that would work, but so far nothing. A few people have recommended that I see a specialist, but I keep thinking I won't need to, that next month I'll be pregnant. What do you think, am I just kidding myself?

It .is very difficult for some couples to acknowledge that they need to see an infertility specialist. Sometimes gynecologists are similarly slow to recognize the need to refer a couple to a reproductive endocrinologist.

According to RESOLVE, a national organization for infertility patients, any of the following situations warrant seeing an infertility specialist:

- couples who are so-called normal infertiles; in other words, those whose basic tests came back normal but who after two years have not yet succeeded in conceiving
- patients who need microsurgery or treatment for endometriosis or tubal damage
- patients with a history of three or more miscarriages
- patients who have irregular menstrual cycles with evidence of irregular ovulation
- patients with poor semen analysis showing a low count, low motility, or poor morphology
- women who are thirty-five years old or older
- women with a previous history of pelvic infection[2]

Since you have been trying to get pregnant for more than two years and are thirty-five, we recommend you move on to a specialist. Who should you see? A number of resources are available to help patients find the right specialist:

There are about 500 Board Certified Reproductive Endocrinologists in the USA. Another 800 plus doctors are Board eligible. It should also be noted that some doctors can also "learn by doing" and are considered to have expertise in infertility. [And] urologists with a sub-speciality called Andrology are the most highly qualified physicians to deal with all aspects of male factor infertility.[3]

These sources can help you find a specialist:

1. Contact the national organization or local chapter of RESOLVE for refer-
    rals to specialists in your area. If possible, go to a meeting of your local chap-
    ter. *Members themselves are the best resource for referrals.* Since all the members are
    consumers of medical care, most of those you talk with have already been to
    a specialist (some more than one) and are familiar with the doctors' treatment,
    styles, office staffs, procedures, fees, and so on. Although you will still have to
    ask many quesitons of the staff and the physician themselves, RESOLVE
    meetings are a good place to start.
2. Your own gynecologist most likely will be able to refer you to a specialist in
    your area.
3. The American Society for Reproductive Medicine has a referral list of their
    members available. (See Appendix II for further information.)

Taking that first step into a specialist's office is never easy, but reassure
yourself that you are doing all you possibly can to reach your goal of creating a
family.

2. How Can I Become a Better Health-Care Consumer?

**My husband is really upset with me because every time he asks me what hap-
pened at the doctor's office, I can't seem to remember. This has never happened to
me before, my memory has always been very good. I start stumbling over my words
when I talk with the doctor. I feel like a fool most times. Is this common?**

Yes, it is very common for infertility patients to have difficulty talking to their
physician and retaining information. Mostly this is because each trip to the doctor's office is fraught with anxiety. What does all the infertility lingo (inseminations, laparoscopies, hysterosalpingograms, and so forth) mean? Will the treatment
hurt? How many tries will it take to get pregnant? No wonder your concentra-
tion level has been compromised. The inability to retain information when you
are in a highly anxious state is a normal response. Most people in a crisis remember information bit by bit, which allows them to get used to the reality of
their situation and at the same time figure out varying ways to cope with the
stress.[4]

You might feel stronger in your relationship with your physician if you follow these guidelines developed by Sidelines, an organization that supports women
who are under incredible amounts of stress due to high-risk pregnancies:[5]

1. *Consider Yourself an Important Member of Your Health-Care Team*   Indicate an interest in knowing all about your situation. Be your own advocate.

2. *Approach Your Physician with Respect and Demand the Same Back*   This means learning to be assertive but not aggressive. Be friendly, straightforward, and respect the doctor's time constraints, while seeing that your own needs are met. Recognize that your doctor is a human being who may have a lot of knowledge about infertility but who is human just the same.

3. *Ask Direct Questions*   One way to counteract the stress is to be ready with written questions before you go to your doctor's appointment. As questions arise in between appointments, jot them down. Then you can simply write the doctor's response next to your prepared questions. Another idea is to bring a tape recorder to the office. If you feel uncomfortable interrupting the conversation with writing, you can tape the conversation and there will be no room for interpretation. If your husband is unable to be present at the appointments, he will be able to get information and answers directly from your doctor.

4. *Express Your Feelings in a Direct but Nonthreatening Way*   "You don't spend enough time with me!" may be better expressed as, "I understand you have a busy schedule, but I feel a need to talk with you at greater length. When would be a convenient time?"

5. *Be Specific*   Just as it is frustrating to hear your doctor say "You are not ovulating" without giving you an explanation, it is equally detrimental for you to give only general descriptions. For instance, if you tell your doctor you feel funny after you take Clomid, he or she might not pay too much attention. But if you are specific, like "I have headaches" or "I am seeing spots before my eyes after I take the medication," the doctor will be more apt to treat you accordingly.

Remember you are the consumer, spending a lot of time and money for this service. You are entitled to get the best care possible.

3. Will My Doctor Reject Me If I Seek a Second Opinion?

I have been working with a good doctor for the past three years. Although I really trust him, my friends have been telling me I should get a second opinion. I'm afraid that if I do, he might not want to see me anymore. And maybe this sounds crazy, but I worry that if he does continue to see me and finds out I've been to another doctor, he'll no longer try very hard to get me pregnant. What should I do?

Think for a minute about other professions. Before submitting any important project or report most people run their findings by at least one colleague to see if there is something they have overlooked. Even in writing this book we consulted many other resources to be sure that our work was as complete as possible. Why then expect doctors to handle treatment plans alone?

Although many of the tests and treatments for infertility are routine, how a doctor interprets these test results and ultimately treats his or her patients is based on experience, training, and instinct. These variables can leave doctors even within the same practice disagreeing on how a patient should proceed. It is important to note, however, that differing opinions do not imply that one physician is right and the other wrong. It simply means that medicine is not the exact science we would like it to be, and that our physicians do not always have the answers we would like them to have. Therefore it is just good common sense to get a second opinion.

Obtaining a second opinion may not be an easy thing to do. Some doctors *will* be put off by their patients' requests. But the majority of doctors routinely consult with other physicians. Conscientious doctors often have to remind their patients that they do not have all the answers. We have to remind ourselves that doctors are not omnipotent.

While getting a second opinion may feel like a big risk, the risk is actually smaller than you think and an important one to take. It would be very sad for you to look back years from now knowing you did not do everything you possibly could to try and get pregnant.

4. Where Can I Find a Therapist Who Specializes in Infertility?

I have been trying to get pregnant for two years, and have been seeing a specialist for one year. I had hoped that by now he would have found something wrong and fixed it. But so far he has no answers and I'm still not pregnant. It's getting harder and harder to be optimistic. Some days all I want to do is cry. I don't really have anyone to talk to about this—all my friends are very fertile. I've been thinking about seeing a therapist just to talk about how I'm feeling, only I'm not sure how to find someone who will understand what I'm going through.

Having someone to talk to about your feelings would probably be a helpful and comforting experience for you at this difficult and often lonely time. Private therapy, couples therapy, or even a support group are all good options:

- Individual therapy provides an opportunity to explore your own feelings and can give you the personalized attention you need to focus in on issues most pressing for you.
- Couples therapy can help you and your husband come to terms with those infertility issues that are having an impact on each of you and on your marriage. Counseling enables couples to gain greater understanding of each other's views and offers them a chance to broaden their communication skills. (See Chapter 3.)
- Support groups offer a chance to see how others handle their infertility and can prepare you for what lies ahead. A support group can also help you feel less alone as you see how much you have in common with the other women.

These options are not mutually exclusive. Many people chose to do more than one at the same time or one right after another.

RESOLVE and the American Society for Reproductive Medicine can assist you in finding a qualified therapist. Their addresses can be found in Appendix II. Locally, your physician or hospital may also be able to refer you to a qualified therapist who works with infertility patients. Support groups for adoption, pregnancy loss, DES, or endometriosis can provide referrals for those who inquire

What if you are locked into an insurance plan that does not include any of the recommended therapists? There are several options. Ask the recommended therapist if he or she would agree to take a lower fee, or consider joining a support group. Most groups are time-limited and less expensive than individual therapy, and leaders are usually willing to work out either a payment schedule or a reduced fee. Or shop around for the best "plan" therapist you can find. Although most people prefer to work with someone who has experienced infertility themselves, the truth is that a therapist with a good background in loss or grief counseling can be equally as helpful with your infertility. While not familiar with the medical procedures, she or he certainly can support you through the emotional ups and downs of the cycle.

Here are some questions to ask when interviewing potential therapists:

1. What are your credentials? (Depending on what state you live in, a therapist may need various licenses or certifications.)
2. What is your training/speciality?

3. How many years of experience have you had as a counselor or therapist?

4. Are you familiar with issues around loss in general and infertility in particular?

5. What is your fee per session, and how long is each session? What insurance do you accept?

6. What are your office hours? Do you work days, evenings, and weekends?

7. Do you charge for time spent on the phone with you?

8. What is your cancellation policy? (Unlike other clients, infertility patients are subject to last-minute, sometimes erratic schedule changes due to the demands of medical treatment. A therapist who charges for these missed appointments would not be a good match for an infertility patient.)

No matter whom you choose, get referrals from reliable sources familiar with the therapists and their work, and shop around until you find someone you are comfortable with.

5. What About the Drugs?

My husband and I have been trying to have a baby for two years. About six months ago we started seeing a specialist. Although she hasn't been able to find anything wrong with either me or my husband, she has just suggested I take Clomid to increase the number of eggs released. She believes this might give me a better chance of getting pregnant. But some of the women in my support group say Clomid has made them feel irritable and just not like themselves. I also keep seeing reports about infertility drugs being linked to various cancers. I really do want to be pregnant, but this is not an easy decision. Do I have any alternatives? Do you have any insights that might help me decide what to do?

When we were infertility patients over ten years ago, we talked about how grateful we were to be experiencing infertility at a time when there were so many medical advances and options available to us. We wondered how people had coped with infertility before the intrauterine inseminations, sonograms, donor inseminations, surgeries, surrogates, and IVF. Thank God for Clomid, Pergonal, Metrodin, Lupron, and Danazol. They would save us; we were sure of it. And when we gave in to the voice of instinct to ask our doctors, "Is it safe?" they couldn't tell us, because they did not know. The government did not care enough to check, really check. Like the women who had taken DES, we had became calculated risks, statistics on a chart in some researcher's office.

Today we are being told by some researchers that we have a higher risk of ovarian cancer than the general population because of some of these drugs. We have also been assured by other researchers that we do not. We have found no clear-cut answers, just a mass of contradictory and confusing reports from those who are objective as well as from those who have a vested interest in seeing these drugs remain on the market.

So in part we are tempted to tell you, "Stop. Don't do it. It's not worth the risk. They don't know if it's safe. Learn from us." But how could we? It would be hypocritical of us. In spite of the risks, we did not want anyone to tell *us* to stop; we did not want to hear the no that would mean no pregnancy and no children. The unknown risks of the drugs were far less threatening to us than the risk of saying no too soon—of letting go before we were ready to look at other options and saying goodbye to that biological child we wanted so desperately.

Ultimately you will have to make the difficult decision of how many cycles (if any) you can risk without jeopardizing your physical and emotional health. Only you can know how far you are willing to travel in order to become pregnant.

We suggest that you look into various alternatives, such as moving to high-tech treatments in a timely manner, thus avoiding many months of drug treatments on low-tech options such as inseminations. Or try an alternative, more natural approach to your infertility as either an adjunct to or a substitute for the high-tech drugs and treatments of today.

One such alternative is naturopathic medicine, which employs many forms of natural treatments in its approach to health care.

> The basic tenet behind naturopathic medicine is to support and strengthen the inherent healing ability of the body specifically the immune system, so it can repair itself. "Do not harm," an oath taken by all physicians, is carried out in the least invasive manner possible using diet, exercise, life-style modification, clinical nutrition, botanicals, homeopathy, physical therapy, hydrotherapy, counseling and other therapies.[6]

Also employed as alternatives to the high-tech treatments of today are various stress reduction techniques, chiropractic care, and acupuncture. (For further information about alternative treatments for infertility, see Appendix II.)

Like all health-care treatments, naturopathic medicines should be approached with as much consideration for their safety and efficacy as you would any medical treatment. This means discussing the practitioner's training, experience with infertility, success rates, procedures, willingness to work with an infertility specialist, and fees. Patients should also inquire about drug interactions, proper use of prescribed herbs, and, "if receiving acupuncture treatment, be certain that disposable needles are used."[7]

Whatever route you decide to take, always ask questions, consider your alternatives, and proceed with caution while keeping in mind your age (how much time you can reasonably afford to spend on any one treatment), your finances, and your ultimate goal.

6. I'm Over Forty—Am I Too Old to Seek Treatment?

My husband and I have been married for three years now. It is a second marriage for both of us. Although my husband has a daughter from his previous marriage, my first husband and I never had any children. I would really like to have a child with my husband, but I have been trying to get pregnant for the past thirteen months, and nothing is happening. At forty-three I don't feel I have a lot of time to waste, so I've made an appointment with a specialist. Now my friends and family think I'm crazy. They say I'm just too old to have a baby and that the kind of treatments I'll need such as IVF will bankrupt us both financially and emotionally. Sometimes I think they're right, but I try to keep their comments out of my mind. Am I just too old?

You are wise to question how your age and your financial and emotional resources will affect your pursuit of pregnancy. Since we live in a world where age does not play as critical a role as it once did in becoming a parent, only you and your husband in consultation with a physician can decide whether there are too many financial, emotional, and medical roadblocks to overcome.

Spontaneous pregnancy success rates drop sharply for women over forty, yet with reproductive assistance success rates increase. From a medical standpoint, it does not seem unreasonable for you to consider treatment. In 1997 an IVF cycle averaged about $9,000 including the fees for drugs, doctors, and hospital services. Usually a couple in your age bracket has to undergo more than one cycle. Other options are donor egg, donor embryo, gestational carrier, and adoption. (See Chapters 9 and 11 for a more thorough discussion of these alternatives.)

It is wise to discuss the emotional reality of infertility treatments and parenthood with your husband. Sometimes the wife in a second marriage feels compelled to have children because of an unspoken and sometimes unconscious competition with her husband's prior marriage, especially if that marriage produced children. Sometimes the second wife presumes that her husband expects her to get pregnant.

However, many times the husband in a second marriage does not want more children. He feels the parenting part of his life is over and is looking forward to a more carefree lifestyle. If you choose to proceed with medical treatment or adoption, make sure you and your husband are clear about each other's feelings and expectations.

7. Infertility Testing Invades My Privacy

My wife and I have recently begun infertility testing. I was asked to give a semen sample to our physician for evaluation. I found the environment in her office to be lacking in privacy. What once was a very personal and private act has been taken into the public arena! I know I have to repeat the test, but what if I can't?

The busy and aseptic atmosphere of your physician's office is hardly an environment conducive to producing a sperm sample. While it may not bother some, most men experience some anxiety. Adding to this stress is the underlying worry about whether the semen is viable. And on top of all this, many wives and physicians expect men to produce the desired sample in a timely manner. The pressure to produce a sample is even greater when an insemination, GIFT *(gamete intrafallopian transfer),* or IVF procedure is involved.

There are a number of ways to deal with your anxiety. First, consider talking with your wife about how you are feeling. Tell her your apprehensions, and ask her for her support and understanding. No doubt she will be able to relate to your feelings since most women have gone through many tests and treatments that are embarrassing or uncomfortable.

Second, speak to your physician about alternative ways to produce semen samples. For instance, if you do not live a great distance from your physician's office or hospital, the sample can be produced at home. It should be produced thirty-six to ninety-six hours after you last ejaculated, and collected in a container supplied by your physician. If you have difficulty masturbating, some physicians say that you can use a nonspermicidal, silicon condom while making love with your wife. Samples can safely be transferred to a medically approved container, then transported in your shirt pocket so it remains warm next to your body. No matter how your sperm is collected, make sure it is brought to the lab within two hours of its retrieval. Because samples vary, a minimum of two specimens should be analyzed. More testing may be necessary if there is a significant variation.[8]

8. Why Is My Husband Having Trouble Accepting Donor Insemination?

My husband had varicocele surgery last year, but it was not successful. His sperm count is still very low. We have tried inseminations where his sperm was washed, but that hasn't worked either. I have really had enough. I want to move on now to donor insemination, but my husband won't hear of it. He says the child should come from both of us or neither of us. I don't understand why he feels this way. Do all husbands have trouble accepting donor insemination?

In theory, donor insemination is a relatively expedient, easy (depending on the wife's fertility), and inexpensive method of creating a family. It would seem, then, to be the perfect solution to a male infertility problem.

However, in order to make this major life decision, the couples we have spoken with felt they needed time to explore their feelings. Some husbands felt the need to go a bit slower than their wives because their self-esteem had been challenged by the diagnosis of male infertility. (See Chapter 1 for a more thorough discussion of male identity.) As one man said,

> When I discovered I was not going to make my wife pregnant, I felt really guilty, like I was really letting her down. I never had any trouble with sex before, so I never expected this. Everyone expects a man to know how to do it. If I were to tell my friends about my infertility, they'd probably make jokes about it and I'd never hear the end of it.

If your husband is experiencing similar feelings, it may be extremely painful for him to imagine your conceiving a baby with another man's sperm. Even though sex is not involved with the donor and the donor will most likely remain anonymous, your husband may have jealous feelings. And, to complicate matters, he might reject these feelings as being irrational, which is why he is not talking to you about them. Your husband may still be coming to terms with his own feelings about being infertile and so may need more time than you to consider donor sperm as a viable parenting option. Remember, up until now your husband has been trying various treatments assuming something would work. Suddenly you are asking him to give up trying to have a biological child, and he might not be ready to do that.

Perhaps it is time for you and your husband to seek out a therapist who specializes in infertility. Even a few sessions can help put the two of you on a path to better understanding. You may also want to seek out other couples who have chosen donor insemination.*

9. Who Should We Ask to Be Our Ovum Donor: Friend, Relative, or Stranger?

My wife and I have decided that our next step will be ovum donation. Our doctor said we could use either an anonymous donor or someone we know. Deciding who to ask is driving us crazy. Should it be a family member, a friend, or a complete stranger? My wife has two married sisters who each would probably be hurt if we asked the other one. Any advice?

Deciding which donor to choose is like looking into a crystal ball to see what your future will hold. In order to make the most informed decision possible, here are some questions for you and your wife to explore:

1. Imagine a child that is genetically related to your sister or sister-in-law:
   What will the child be like?
   What will the child look like?
   How important is that genetic continuity to you?
2. Imagine the child from a friend or an unknown donor:
   How will you feel if the child does not look like either you or your wife?
3. *(For your wife:)* Imagine what it will feel like to carry a fetus formed by . . .
   your husband and your sister;
   your husband and a friend;
   your husband and an unknown donor.
4. Imagine telling your child about his or her origins. How does that feel?
5. Imagine watching your child interacting with a friend or family member as donor. What role will she play? Specifically:
   How much influence will you feel comfortable having the donor exert in your child's life?
   What if the donor does not agree with your parenting style?
6. Imagine having a conversation with your family or friends about your plans:
   How comfortable would you be telling them about your choice of donor?

---

* For an in-depth discussion of the details of donor insemination, see Susan L. Cooper and Ellen S. Glazer, *Beyond Infertility: The New Pathways to Parenthood* (Lexington Books, New York, 1994), pp. 138–196.

Would you tell other family members that your sister or sister-in-law is the baby's donor?

If you decide on using a donor from your family, you can ask both sisters to help you make the decision. One may opt out on her own. However, if both are interested in being a donor, they can be evaluated by the professional staff at your clinic. Each sister's fertility status, marital relationship (your brothers-in-law should also be consulted), and general medical and psychological condition will be assessed. In addition, the clinic will explore your relationship with your siblings to determine how they will feel once the baby is born and part of the family.

If you decide on an unknown donor, your clinic will provide you with a list of applicants. (Since the procedure is so physically and emotionally taxing, egg donors are not as readily available as sperm donors.) Make sure the donor has been well screened medically and counseled about the emotional aspects of donating her ova.

It is important for you and your wife to approach your decision with tender loving care. If done with perseverance and respect for one another as well as for the donor and your future baby, you may have the opportunity to experience the long-awaited joy of pregnancy and parenthood.★

10. Should We Consider Gestational Care—Having Another Woman Carry Our Baby?

My wife is infertile. Although her ovaries can produce eggs, she can't carry a pregnancy to term. We're thinking about having a baby who would be genetically ours but "grown" in a surrogate's body. We read about the idea in a magazine. What are the legal and medical implications, and where can we find someone willing to be a surrogate?

Gestational care, a term coined by Susan Cooper and Ellen Glazer in their book, *Beyond Infertility,* is described as being somewhat similar to traditional surrogacy, in that the baby is grown in another woman's body. The difference is that the baby would genetically come from both you and your wife, whereas in traditional surrogacy the baby would derive from you (the male) and the female surrogate.

Also different is the fact that the gestational carrier's emotional attachment to

★ For a thorough discussion of the issues surrounding ovum donation, we highly recommend Cooper and Glazer's book, *Beyond Infertility,* pp. 197–259.

the child seems to be less strong. According to a group of infertility specialists from Pennsylvania Reproductive Associates,

> The importance of genetic distinction has been reaffirmed through clinical experience. Women evaluated as potential gestational carriers report that they can accept carrying a child that is biologically unrelated to them and they feel that they would have great emotional difficulty relinquishing a child that is, in part, biologically theirs. Being genetically inert, the carriers report that they are able to separate themselves emotionally from the baby and decrease the attachment process throughout the pregnancy.[9]

This emotional separation might not always translate into the parents' control of the baby's health while the carrier is pregnant. Do the baby's genetic parents have the right to tell the carrier what to eat and drink, which doctor to see, and what medicines to take? These issues need to be sorted out ahead of time and perhaps incorporated into a legal contract.[10]

Once the baby is born, a legal agreement needs to be in place to guarantee the genetic parents their rights to the child. This is handled in different ways by gestational care programs. Some lawyers file maternity and paternity suits on behalf of the genetic parents prior to the delivery of the child. Since the gestational carrier is not interested in parenting the baby, the genetic parents' rights go uncontested by her. Other lawyers have found similar ways to petition the courts to guarantee parental rights. With the exception of one case in 1990, where the gestational mother filed for parental rights (she was not awarded the child), there has been little contesting of the legal arrangements made between gestational carriers and genetic parents intending to raise the child.[11]

As Coleen Friedman, C.S.W., a specialist in infertility practicing in Chicago, says, "Any couple who is going to enter into this kind of arrangement with a gestational carrier needs to be aware that because this sort of relationship is so new, there are issues that will come up that none of us can foresee."[12] If you are interested in this method, there are organizations listed in Appendix II that might be able to help you.

11. Sometimes Medical Treatment Feels Like Rape

I may be the only person on the planet who feels this way, but I am having a lot of trouble going to the doctor for infertility treatments. I was raped when I was in high school, in what they now call date rape, but back then I just thought it was my fault and told absolutely no one. I carried around a lot of guilt for a long time, but after much hard work in therapy, I felt I had put it behind me. But sometimes when I go to the doctor the memories of that night come back to me, and then I find it really hard to make love to my husband. This isn't exactly the kind of thing you can bring up at a RESOLVE meeting. Am I crazy?

No, you are not. In her book *Men, Women and Infertility,* Aline P. Zoldbrod has a chapter entitled "Medical Treatment as Rape" in which she acknowledges that women with a history of sexual abuse, rape, or battering may be at even higher risk of having sexual problems following infertility treatment than other patients. As Zoldbrod explains,

> The woman who is on the doctor's examining table, feet in stirrups, about to ex-
> perience physical pain in the genital region at the hands of the physician, who
> is standing above her, is in a situation filled with the signs and signals of domi-
> nance, submission, and a subtle message of threat. . . . This is a situation of great
> vulnerability for the patient, even if she doesn't recognize the fact. . . . [One
> woman reported that] During a procedure, she had told her physician to stop be-
> cause she was in such pain, and his only response was to continue to do what he
> was doing, only faster.[12]

Other women have reported that infertility was the final blow to a sex life already severely damaged by previous rape or abuse experiences.

Some of the techniques described in Appendix I may help you to separate your lovemaking from your medical and rape experience. Consider going back to some of the techniques you may have learned during your previous therapy and see if you can apply them to your current situation. Sharing with your husband what is going on for you also may take some of the pressure off. Also consider going back to your previous therapist if possible or finding a new one who is experienced in both loss and abuse issues.

At present you need support for your feelings and help in coping with your day-to-day infertility issues. Infertility in of itself can be damaging, but infertility on top of a previously abusive experience can be truly devastating, and support can make all the difference in the world.

12. I'm Afraid of Early Menopause

I am only thirty-two years old, and last week the second doctor I have seen for a consultation about my infertility told me I'm starting menopause. But I keep thinking I will go home and there will be a message from the doctor's office telling me that the test results were incorrect and I am fine. I'm scared and very confused about what to do next.

Hearing you are going through menopause is a shock. Give yourself some time to emotionally absorb what this means to you and the losses this experience carries with it.

You will also want to look at menopause from a medical standpoint. You may be surprised to discover that many of your assumptions about menopause are not correct. For example, "menopause will make you old before your time." This outdated, frightening belief comes from a time when menopause was misunderstood, misdiagnosed, and mistreated. "Thanks to the new reproductive technologies, premature menopause does not have to mean a premature end to the reproductive years. With hormonal priming and donor eggs, postmenopausal women—particularly those under forty-five—may still be capable of carrying out a pregnancy."[14]

We suggest you learn more about the complexities of menopause by researching books and articles and by asking your doctor for further information. See Appendix II for resources.

7

Working Through Loss
Coping with Grief and Mourning

Ashes settle on velvet skin
caressed by the blood of birth
left in the field of tall beige grass
a funeral attended by nature
as birds gather to talk of this tiny body
fallen into their midst
meant to be, meant to be
they cried into the wind
and the words swirled into the air
into human minds
that took in this song as their own
only to be whispered out
at funerals, in hospital corridors, in morgues
mourners and doctors, the ones left behind
ease their pain
console their hearts
wipe their tears
by repeating the song of the birds
meant to be, meant to be
Challenged by no one, carried across the land
across the sea, across time
the grieving inhale these words
with every breath, repeat them
throw them up
to the wind, so all might catch them,
catch them, take them as if always owned
meant to be, meant to be
And no one questioned
no one asked
how they knew
what if not
what if
what if
it was not
meant to be, not meant to be.
What if the birds were wrong
what if that baby's death was not meant to be.
                              —Debby Peoples

Grief is not quicksand.
Rather, it is a walk on rocky terrain
that eventually smooths out and provides less challenge—
both emotionally and physically.
                    —Carol Staudacher, *Men and Grief*[1]

The losses we discuss in this chapter are painful. Those of you who have suffered the loss of a child through miscarriage, adoption loss,[*] ectopic pregnancy, still birth, early delivery, or multifetal pregnancy reduction will relate to the pain and frustration of each of the following couples as they struggle with the intensity of their grief. This chapter of the book has been one of the most difficult to write because we know how inadequate words on a page or even the spoken word can be when you are in the depths of grief.

The emotions that accompany grief may be so overpowering that, at times, it may seem they will never go away. Grief can be very scary. It is like being at the bottom of an ocean and trying to swim to the surface for air before losing your breath. Like being underwater, everything becomes blurred and nothing is clear. Places you have gone to and things you have done countless times before seem strangely unfamiliar—even colors may appear to have changed. The pressure and stress can be enormous. You may find yourself experiencing a sadness so deep you cannot even imagine where it is coming from or how to make it go away. Your arms long to hold your baby. Your fingers crave to touch the softness of your baby's skin. You may have thought that infertility was the worst thing that could happen to you, but now you have found something worse. Although infertility involves many losses, it is a crisis that builds slowly over time. The loss of a baby, on the other hand, usually happens relatively quickly, without warning, and shakes your very foundation. And although pregnancy and adoption losses are in some ways differ-

---

[*] *Adoption loss* is when a birth parent changes his or her mind prior to or after placement of the child with the adoptive parents, at which point the birth parents either maintain custody or regain custody of the child through the courts.

  Because the information available to us on this subject was so limited, we conducted our own research. We spoke with many couples on an informal basis from New York to California. In addition we formally surveyed fourteen couples gracious enough to share their stories about how and when the babies they fell in love with were taken away from them. We were struck by the silence surrounding both the prevalence of adoption loss and the deep sadness that accompanies it.

ent, each carries with it the same emotional pain. Grief and healing is a slow, mournful process.

Grief is different for each individual. It runs its own course with no time limits or set stages. Grief envelops and invades who you are, and what you have lost now and in the past. In *Motherless Daughters: The Legacy of Loss,* Hope Edelman describes what she learned about grief after losing her mother: "It's not linear. It's not predictable. It's anything but smooth and self-contained. Someone did us a grave injustice by first implying that mourning has a distinct beginning, middle, and end. That's the stuff of short fiction. It's not real life." Later she talks about the inappropriateness of time limitations for grief: "We're an impatient culture accustomed to gratifying most of our needs quickly. But mourning requires a certain resignation to the forces of time. Expecting grief to run a quick, predictable course has led us to overpathologize the process, viewing normal responses as indicators of serious distress."[2]

Although there are no set rules or time limits for grieving, there are many common reactions to loss. Below is a list of these loss reactions so that you can clearly see that your experiences are a natural part of the grieving and healing process. Some of you will relate to almost all of these experiences, others to just a few. The number of items you respond to however, will have little to do with the longevity or intensity of your pain.

Typical Reactions to Loss[3]

- shock/numbness
- crying
- feeling crazy
- disinterest in sex
- feeling very alone
- denial
- feeling out of control
- intense sadness
- lethargy
- jealousy
- marital friction
- moving toward or away from religion or spirituality
- blaming God, spouse, doctor, environment, lawyers—anyone perceived to be at fault

- grief-related feelings that may return around the anniversary date of the birth or loss of the baby
- avoidance of children and/or couples who have children—particularly of children born when your child was or should have been born
- trying to occupy all your free time
- feeling like you want to die.★
- nightmares and/or insomnia
- depression
- shortness of breath
- confusion
- fear of of being alone
- anger
- tightening in your chest and throat
- forgetfulness
- stress
- guilt
- feelings of emptiness and longing
- feelings of failure and embarrassment
- reliving the event over and over again
- an increase or decrease in appetite
- physical symptoms, such as hormonal changes, headaches, stomach distress, backaches
- preoccupation with thoughts about the child and/or events leading up to the loss
- a strong need to be reclusive (alone)

Reactions Specific to Pregnancy Loss

- body and hormonal changes specific to pregnancy as a constant reminder of your loss
- anger and/or or mistrust of the medical community including physicians, nurses, office and hospital staff, and so on.

★ While the intensity of the grief makes many men and women feel their world has come to an end, it is not a symptom to be taken lightly. If you feel this way, tell someone, preferably a clergy person or therapist, who can help you get through this very difficult time.

Reactions Specific to Adoption Loss

- general mistrust of the world
- fantasies of failed future adoption situations
- mistrust of any or all of the following: birth mothers and birth fathers, lawyers, therapists, agencies, and the legal systems of the United States and other countries
- fantasies of a failed adoption being reversed and the birth mother returning the baby to the adoptive parents

In addition to the effects of loss on an individual, loss deeply affects most marriages. "The death of a child has a paradoxical effect on the relationship between the parents. The shared loss creates a new and very profound tie between them at the same time that the individual loss each of them feels creates an estrangement in the relationship."[4] This estrangement is often intensified by the dissimilar ways in which men and women approach grief. Generally, men perceive their wives' reactions as being too intense; they may try to get their wives to "stop obsessing" by suggesting involvement in other things besides mourning. Some men try to avoid their wives' grief altogether by working late or finding excuses to leave the house. Still other men see their wives' reactions as being pathological (like an illness) and may suggest antidepressant drugs, even when their wives' grief is completely within the normal and expected range.

Women, on the other hand, tend to monitor their husbands' grief reaction and judge how much their husbands loved or wanted the child based on how much they discuss their grief or how much they cry after the loss. If husbands do not show their feelings, wives may interpret their reactions as insensitive, unloving, and even cold-hearted. Such inaccurate judgments can leave women feeling angry, frustrated, and even more alone.

Men and women need to remember that outward expressions of grief are not necessarily a gauge of true feelings, as the example below indicates:

After a miscarriage Larry begins to feel sad while watching a baseball game. He dreamed of one day sharing his favorite sport with the child he lost. As the sadness increases, he may work to direct his thoughts elsewhere. He might turn off the television, leave the house, begin working on a project, or take a drive. He feels compelled to take his mind off his sadness.

His wife, Connie, might experience her own sadness on the same day when she opens the mail and finds an invitation to a baby shower. Thinking about the shower she dreamed of having for her own baby, she may begin to cry or feel low for all or part of the day. Eventually she may choose to reach out to a friend for comfort.

At the end of the day, Larry probably won't share what happened to him while he watched the baseball game. Connie may never know how much her husband misses his child. Connie is much more likely to tell her husband about the invitation and how upset she is. At which point Larry will be forced to deal with her feelings. Larry may then come to the conclusion that her feelings are more important than his. Or, he may resent the fact that she brought up the feelings he is trying to avoid. This scenario leaves little room for valuable communication.

While some of the reason for this misunderstanding lies with our cultural expectations for men and women, husbands and wives are, in some very real ways, grieving two different losses. The husband grieves for what the baby would have meant to him, and the wife grieves for what her baby would have meant to her. *Grieving is a personal process.* Alla Renée Bozarth, in her book *Life Is Goodbye, Life Is Hello,* discusses why this is so:

The key is in the meaning which a person invests in what has been given up or taken away by fate, circumstance, or will. In other words, the more someone or something means to me, the more of myself I have invested, given over or entrusted outside of myself. In being cut off from that someone or something, I am in fact cut off from that part of me that the other represented. I have lost a part of my own self. . . . The greater the significance of the now lost person or thing, the more one is likely to believe "I can't be happy without . . ." or even "I can't feel whole without . . ." that other. In extremely painful loss—the kind which might indeed be "deplorable" or even "atrocious" to the sufferer—one may feel and actually believe "I can't live without. . . ." All of these statements really mean "I can't express a part of myself without. . . ."[5]

No matter what loss you have suffered or what your grieving style is, grief cannot be forced or denied. Carol Staudacher outlines the importance of grieving in her book *Men & Grief:*

The reason for processing grief is not to weaken life, but to strengthen it. While the experience of grief is debilitating at the time, such a condition is temporary. To express normal grief—grief that is not inhibited, delayed or distorted in some way—is to work toward a positive life. It makes possible healthful living, instead of a diminished, struggling existence. In fact, grief that is *not* dealt with may very well be debilitating for the rest of the survivor's life. . . . When any survivor's grief is inhibited, delayed or absent, some aspect of his or her life is negatively affected. For example, such a survivor, regardless of gender, is more prone to have an impaired immune-system response, depression, and sleep, appetite, and weight disturbances, as well as an increased mortality risk. With some survivors there will also be a tendency toward drug or alcohol dependence, antisocial behavior, delinquent activity or sexual dysfunction.[6]

Another sign of delayed grief can be an "anniversary reaction." Holidays, the date of the loss, or due dates can bring up an intensity of sadness either equal to or greater than the initial reactions to the loss. This resurgence of emotion may be confusing to people who thought they had "gotten over those feelings." As upsetting as anniversary reactions can be, however, they can be seen as an opportunity to further delve into the unresolved feelings of your loss. For some who did not know how or were unable to deal with their loss initially, an anniversary reaction allows them to revisit the feelings and work through them.[7]

By acknowledging what you have lost and processing the feelings, the negative consequences of unresolved grief can be avoided. Give yourself time alone to think about the baby you have lost. For those who have suffered a loss in which the baby was not actually seen, this may not be easy. However, whether you held your baby or not, name, "see," and memorialize your child. The more tangible you can make your loss, the more completely you can grieve. Some people find it helpful to employ the imagery techniques described in Appendix I, but most people prefer to work with a therapist who specializes in grief. One woman who lost a baby through an ectopic pregnancy shared the images that helped her say goodbye:

> I saw my baby full-term even though she was only weeks old when I lost her. I kept seeing her little lifeless body just lying there. It was horrible, I cried so hard. All I wanted to do was pick her up, but no matter how hard I tried I couldn't. Through my tears I prayed, and an angel soon appeared, picked my baby up, and cradled her in her arms. At that very moment I knew her tiny soul would be taken care of. I still felt a terrible loss, but over time these images brought me comfort and helped me to let her go.

While focusing on the child you lost can be difficult, even painful, it can also be the first step on the long road to recovering from your loss.

Once you have started working through your grief, you will soon find that you do not feel bad every minute of every day. As the days and months pass, you will get longer and longer respites from your pain, and you will begin to feel your energy return. Eventually you will be able to talk about your baby without crying or feeling depressed. You will even find yourself returning to some of the activities you once enjoyed and may start making plans for another child.

1. I'm Afraid of Getting Pregnant Again after Two Miscarriages

I have been trying to have a baby for over four years now. Last year, I finally got pregnant. I was so happy I told practically everyone I saw, even perfect strangers. A month later I lost the baby. I cried for a solid week. Breaking the news to all our friends was so difficult. It took months before I was able to talk about it without tears. I felt so stupid for believing that our infertility was over.

As soon as I started feeling better, we began treatment again. This time I got pregnant right away. I wasn't at all excited because I knew it could be gone in a minute. I thought if I could get past the first month, which was when I had miscarried last time, I would feel better. As each month passed I became a little less anxious. And then it happened—in the fourth month. I'll never forget my obstetrician's words: "I'm not hearing a heartbeat." I only remember the nurse calling my husband to come get me. After that, everything was a blur. I lost the baby a few days later. From that point on, I did only the things people told me to do. I cried and cried. This loss hurt me in a way I have never been hurt before. It took months before I could go to the mall, with all those babies and pregnant women parading around.

My doctor and my husband think I should try once more, but I am terrified of going through another miscarriage.

After enduring years of infertility, it is particularly painful to suffer the loss of both your babies. The deep devastation you felt after your second miscarriage was probably heightened by the length of time you carried, your previous loss and your infertility.

Like infertility, pregnancy loss is another "out of control" situation. No matter how hard you may have tried to take care of yourself, ultimately the circumstances of each of your pregnancies were out of your control. Understandably you are reluctant to put yourself in this vulnerable position again.

Although your husband and doctor are encouraging you to try to get pregnant, wait until *you* are ready. Even though you are feeling better, take some extra time now to heal emotionally and physically before heading back to the strain of another pregnancy. After two losses, the level of stress during your third pregnancy is likely to increase significantly.

Talk to your husband about your fears and concerns. Even if he doesn't share them, he should still be made aware of how you feel. Listen carefully to his reasons for wanting to try again. While you may be focusing on your fears about what will happen if you have another miscarriage, your husband may be focusing on his hope for a successful pregnancy, which in reality is quite high. "If a woman has lost three previous pregnancies without a specific identifiable cause, she still has a 70 to 80 percent chance of carrying a fetus to viability."[8]

If, after your talk, you and your husband still don't agree on when and whether you should try and get pregnant again, we suggest that the two of you pick a mutually agreeable date, preferably at least six months into the future, to both discuss and reevaluate your decisions. This will give you the time you need to get away from the pressure of trying to make a decision you believe you are really not ready to make right now.

During those six months, you might seek out the support of other couples who have experienced both infertility and miscarriage. Talking to these men and women will help you gain support for your feelings and knowledge about pregnancy loss. (A list of these organizations can be found in Appendix II.) If there is no group in your area, ask your physician if he can put you in touch with some women with experiences similar to yours. You can also find support by reading books on miscarriage listed in the Bibliography.

Consider looking for a therapist who can help you sort out your feelings about a future pregnancy. If you do decide to get pregnant again, your therapist will be there through all the uncertainties that are bound to arise. Look for a therapist who specializes in loss issues. Most support organizations will be able to refer you to a qualified professional. Recognize also that if you do get pregnant again, you will feel stress and worry. This is a normal condition for those who have had multiple miscarriages.

The decision ahead of you is a difficult one. However, through open communication with your husband, sharing your experiences with others and working through your feelings with a therapist, you will be more prepared for whatever lies ahead.

2. How Do We Cope with an Adoption Loss?

After five years of infertility, my husband and I chose independent adoption and began advertising eight months ago. None of the many prospective birth mothers

seemed like they would work out, until Jill called us. She was young, unmarried, and said motherhood wouldn't mix with college life; she had plans to return to school as soon as the baby was born. We knew that our prayers were finally being answered. Even our lawyer felt this was a good situation. We talked to Jill once a week and really had a nice phone relationship with her. She was sweet and smart—everything we could have asked for in a birth mother.

Still, the two months of waiting began to feel as long as the five years of our infertility. We did everything we could to keep ourselves busy and our minds off the baby. A part of us kept saying, "Hold on," she could still change her mind.

When the call finally came from Jill's mother that she had just given birth to a boy, we immediately made plane reservations for the next day, and then called everyone we knew to share our wonderful news. My mother cried when I told her, and my sister set a date for a baby shower. Then we were off to the store to stock up on diapers, formula, a car seat, and a few blue outfits. When we got home, our lawyer called to tell us Jill had changed her mind, and would be keeping her baby. We were shocked and confused. That was our baby. Why would she do this? Then we started hoping she would change her mind again, but she never did.

It's been three months since this happened, and we are still devastated. Sometimes we are angry, but mostly we are sad. No one ever explained why she changed her mind or how she was going to take care of the baby. We worry about him.

We are trying to pick ourselves up and start advertising again, but it's been so difficult. All the books we read tell us how to adopt, but none tell us what do when a birth mother changes her mind. How have other people coped with this, and how did they get the strength to go back and try again?

The loss you have suffered is devastating. It is a *real* loss that happens to many couples. Although you did not carry your baby physically, you carried him in your minds and hearts. Like all prospective parents, you probably began bonding with your son prior to his birth. You imagined taking care of him—feeding, changing, rocking—and introducing him to your friends and family. Telling people and buying things for the baby make everything feel more real. Naturally you began to see this baby as your own. Your son represented a hope and a dream. Even if you go on to adopt another baby, there will always be a place in your heart for that child.

Give yourself time to grieve before you move on. The process of grieving for a child who was taken from you in this way can be difficult, because most people associate grief with death. The typical rituals of mourning, such as funerals, are not afforded to those who suffer adoption loss even though such observances can be very helpful. In Chapter 8 we have included information on ways to honor your loss and remember your child. Planning and participating in a ritual may help to direct and process your feelings and to ease your pain.

Recognize also that your concerns for the future of your child are valid. The birth mother convinced you that she had neither the means nor the desire to care for a baby at this point in her life. However, she may not have been able to imagine herself as a parent before she gave birth. It is possible that upon his arrival, she began loving him so much that is was easier to find a way to raise him than to deal with the grief of losing him. While your son will not have the life you could have provided, you may sleep better if you can look at the birth mother's decision as a loving one.

Viewing the birth mother's decision in a positive light does not invalidate your pain or excuse her lack of consideration. You spoke with Jill once a week for over two months and had a relationship on the phone that must have seemed very close. You were going to share something special together. She was about to bestow the greatest gift one can give and you were going to be entrusted to take care of this gift forever. That's not casual conversation. Calling off an adoption through a telephone message relayed by a lawyer may offer the birth mother an easy way out, but unfortunately it leaves the prospective adoptive parents with a lot of unanswered questions and unfinished business. You needed a chance to tell her how you feel.

It's very important for those who have suffered an adoption loss to have some communication with the birth mother and/or birth father. We understand from our interviews with other couples who have suffered adoption losses that it was very enlightening and healing to actually hear the birth mother's voice as she explains why she changed her mind. However, if this is not possible, another alternative is to express your feelings by writing a letter to her, which you may or may not send. This will help put some closure on a situation that can be devastating if it remains open.

Because you have decided to try again to adopt, you will have to deal with the issue of trust. After an adoption loss, the vast majority of couples report that they were unable to trust any future birth parents. Most couples describe their level of trust the next time as being almost nonexistent, and they approached every new situation with caution and extreme scepticism. Some couples coped by doing things differently the second time, some refused private adoption altogether and decided to work with an agency, others switched lawyers, some went out of the country to adopt a child, and still others looked for birth mothers in states that allowed the birth parents the shortest waiting periods for changing their minds.

Regardless of what strategies you employ the second time, the wait for your child will most likely be difficult. To cope with the waiting as well as the fears and the grief that remained, many of the couples we spoke with turned to counseling.

Some sought out a qualified therapist or a support group, while others turned to their clergy. The majority of couples felt better keeping busy with work and vacations or by focusing all their attention on getting another adoption situation. Most couples we spoke to said that even though this waiting period was difficult, they were able to learn and grow from their loss during this time. Many believed that if they had not suffered the loss of their first child, they never would have had the opportunity to adopt their second child.

3. After Losing a Child, Is Getting Pregnant the Answer?

Every doctor visit made my pregnancy feel more real and as each month passed my fantasies of life with my baby grew. But one day I noticed some fluid that I had never seen before. It wasn't very much, so I dismissed it. I figured I had just been on my feet too much that day and promised myself to take it easier from then on.

The next morning I awoke to a pool of fluid on my bed, and no rationalizing could make me believe that everything was okay. The doctor told me to meet him at the hospital right away. There he explained that our daughter would soon be born. At twenty-three weeks there was nothing they could do to save her. We vacillated back and forth between incredible sadness and our own fantasy that the doctor would be proven wrong.

Holding our baby and watching her slowly die in our arms was like being tortured. Here she was, the little girl I had dreamed about for so long, and we had no time to get to know each other. The weeks that followed were a blur in which I barely held myself together. Sometimes I would stop crying long enough to get mad at the doctors or God for not doing something to save my baby. Other times I would take the blame for my daughter's death—if only I had rested more or called the doctor when I first saw the fluid.

It's been two months since my daughter's death, I still don't sleep well. I have nightmares, and I hardly eat anything. My husband says I spend too much time crying. Last week I finally went back to work, only to find that the job I once loved means nothing to me now. Some people are telling me I will feel better if I get pregnant again right away. Others say I need to give myself time. At this point I'd do anything to make this pain go away and get on with my life. Will getting pregnant really help me do that?

One of the most difficult things we face as humans is the loss of a child. As Regina Sara Ryan explains in her book *No Child in My Life,*

Grieving takes time, more time than we think we have and definitely more time than we want to spend. Part of the grief-denying culture is the pervasive message that things can be "fixed," and fast. But when we suffer the loss of child, there is no such thing as instant relief. Nevertheless, the pressures all around us keep encouraging us to settle into business as usual. Some people offer us easy solutions, but what they are really doing is asking us to feel better so that we won't disturb their lives any more. They hurt with us and for us, and they don't like that.[9]

Those friends and relatives encouraging you to get pregnant again quickly are probably having difficulty watching you suffer. They might be the same people who encouraged and applauded your efforts to return to work. But as you have discovered, going back to work did not make the intense sadness go away, even though it may have caused it to abate for brief periods of time. Your eating and sleeping habits, especially your dreams, are clear indications that you are still grieving. "We may be able to paint the clouds silver, but our dreams will show them more starkly grey than ever; dreams tell only the truth and can be tormenting if we deny the truth when we are awake."[10]

Having another child will not make things better or lessen your grief. Just like returning to work, another child may serve to occupy your mind for brief periods of time, but the grief will still be there and the work will have to be done eventually. "In fact, the more pain is denied, the deeper it tends to go inside our bodies and souls, and the harder it is to identify and deal with and ultimately grow beyond.... [T]he only way to get through something is to get *through* it—not over, under, or around it, but all the way through it. And it has to take as long as it takes."[11]

4. IVF Didn't Give Me a Baby

My husband was very reluctant to go through IVF. It took me almost a year to convince him, but when he finally agreed, he said we would have to stop at two cycles, mainly for financial reasons. During my first cycle none of my eggs fertilized. The second cycle was much better: we made it all the way through and transferred three embryos.

I was as close to pregnant as I had ever been. Prior to this, every month was a maybe, but this was different, this was so real. Inside me were three potential babies, and I prayed for every one of them. I even fantasized about what life would be like with triplets. It's not that I didn't know things could go wrong. But this was the first treatment that ever "worked," and I guess I just wanted to believe everything would be okay.

I waited for that phone call to tell me whether I was pregnant or not. It's the weirdest feeling, one minute you believe you could be, and the next minute they're telling you you're not. When I heard the nurse's words, I didn't want to believe them. At first I thought, "No way, this can't be happening." All at once my body felt different, empty, as if life had drained out of me. I was back to nothing. I had lost all my babies.

I have been crying for weeks. Everyone thinks I'm crazy. They don't understand why I'm so upset. "After all," they say, "this isn't the first treatment that's failed, and besides, you weren't really pregnant." I'm beginning to think they are right. But I can't stop thinking about my babies.

Losses can be scary because of the intensity of the feelings that accompany them. Sometimes when we don't "expect" to feel so much, we tend to look at our reactions as abnormal. If someone confirms these fears by telling us we are overreacting, we suffer needless anxiety over what was actually an appropriate response. In our society many people put a limit on how much we should or should not grieve, depending on what we have lost. In your case, however, those judging your grief most likely have never been though infertility. They cannot understand your disappointment and deep sadness over having to end treatment. If you were to meet a group of women with similar experiences, you would find that they understand and share your feelings.

A period of grief would follow this type of loss under any circumstances. However, your reaction is intensified because this was to be your last IVF cycle, and thus the last possibility of ever getting pregnant through medical intervention. Your loss had both a physical component and emotional component. The physical part was the loss of your three fertilized ova which were placed inside you but unable to grow. You physically held them in your body. They were real. The emotional component is difficult for others to comprehend and for you to deal with because it is so intangible. It encompasses all the fantasies taken away when you found out you were not pregnant this time, and all the times before. You are losing the dream of maternity clothes, a baby shower, a nursery, toys, breast feeding, maybe a christening or a naming, family gatherings, play dates—all the joys of motherhood you wanted so badly. You *have lost* three babies in a very real way. If you *do* stop mourning the loss of these children you wanted so desperately, you will do yourself a great disservice.

This is a time in which you can mourn your losses and "explore your options" so that eventually you will be able to look ahead to the future. The suggestions offered in this chapter can help you get in touch with your true feelings. Then you will be better able decide whether to save more money and try IVF again, look into adoption, or think about child-free living—all valid choices which you will want to consider. Chapter 9 will give you further insight into this decision-making process.

5. Should We Try Again or Remain Child-Free?

We had unexplained infertility and tried for six years to have a baby. We went through every test and treatment, spent thousands of dollars, and still had no baby. After many painful discussions we decided to live child-free. Although there were days in our new lifestyle when we missed having a child, we were relieved not to have to deal with the infertility anymore. For two years we used our savings for travel and hobbies instead of infertility drugs and treatments. We found a new circle of friends; some of whom were child-free, and others who had grown children with a lot of free time to spend with friends.

Then out of the clear blue, my wife got pregnant. In spite of our comfort with child-free living, we immediately found ourselves excited over the possibility of becoming parents. We made plans to convert the study to a nursery and canceled our upcoming trip, as we could no longer afford to spend our money on travel. During the next few months we continued to make new plans and cancel old ones. Then it happened: a miscarriage. We were not prepared, the rug had once again been pulled out from under us, and we were left with nothing.

Our doctor encouraged us to try again. Although we have talked about it over and over, we can't decide what to do. My wife is terrified of another pregnancy, and we were really getting comfortable with our child-free lifestyle. On the other hand, the thought of becoming parents made us very happy at the time. Any suggestions for resolving our dilemma?

Losing a child to miscarriage is difficult under any circumstances. On top of that you have had to endure a roller-coaster lifestyle of infertility, child-free living, fertility, and then back to infertility. A pregnancy after a couple has settled into a child-free lifestyle does not carry the same meaning as during their infertility. Most child-free couples, when faced with an unexpected pregnancy, find they have very mixed feelings about becoming parents.

Couples who subsequently lose the pregnancy have even more to deal with as they must mourn the loss of their child, revisit their old infertile feelings, and decide where to go next. This visit back to the decision-making process is where you are right now. You sound as if you are feeling pressured to come up with an answer about what to do next. Perhaps you feel you must decide quickly, before whatever got "fixed" enough to allow for pregnancy "breaks" again. More likely though, this return to infertility is so disconcerting that you are desperate to resolve it in order to get your lives back on track.

Whatever is pushing you, remember the reasons for your original child-free decision. The decision you now face is not much different. Yes, you will have to consider the fact that your wife got pregnant, but you will also have to think about what it would feel like to go back again full-time to overcoming infertility. You may find, to your surprise that it would no longer be worth it to put yourself through the stress and anxiety of trying to go after and keep another pregnancy. At this point, the prospect of putting your life on hold again may be too much to bear.

If age is not an overriding factor in your decision-making process, we suggest that you and your wife consider going back to a child-free lifestyle for a while. A year off will allow you to find out what is right for you in a less pressured way. After your decision, don't be surprised if you experience brief periods of grieving again for whatever lifestyle you have decided to give up. After all major life decisions there are times of feeling unsure; this is a necessary part of moving on not a sign of having made the wrong choice. Expect this uneasiness to occur, and remember to keep it in perspective.

If you do decide to live child-free, we urge you to start using some form of birth control (providing it does not conflict with your religious or moral beliefs). Although it may seem strange to use contraception after years of infertility, many couples report that not having to worry about pregnancy each month helped them to put their infertility in the past. (See Chapter 10 for further discussion on lifestyle changes.)

By taking the time to rest and regroup, you should find the answer you seek. Hindsight can sometimes shed the brightest light. Good luck.

6. Was My Ectopic Pregnancy a Real Loss?

A week after I made my first appointment with an infertility specialist, I found out I was pregnant. At the time I didn't know why it had taken me two years to get pregnant, but the day the stick turned blue, I no longer cared. All the anxiety disappeared as I suddenly became "normal" again. It felt so great to be pregnant after wanting it for so long.

The first few weeks were relatively uneventful except for some periodic abdominal pain, which my doctor dismissed. In the fifth week the pain increased and finally got so bad I ended up in the emergency room. There I was diagnosed with an ectopic pregnancy. The doctor told me I had to have surgery immediately, that waiting could kill me. The IVs were put in, and I was prepped for surgery. My husband held my hand. My feelings were coming at me from every direction. I didn't want to lose my baby, but I didn't want to die. After the surgery my doctor told me that although he had had to remove one of my tubes, he'd also saved my life. I looked at my doctor as a sort of hero. After all, thanks to him I was alive. It has taken me months to realize that the opposite is really the truth. Because he kept ignoring my complaints, he had actually almost killed me.

It has also taken me months to realize that I lost a baby. I know this sounds ridiculous, but everyone has been so caught up in the surgery, the loss of my tube, and the recovery process that no one ever mentioned the baby. People only want to know how soon we can try again. The problem is, I am scared I will have another ectopic pregnancy. Even my husband doesn't want me to try again, because he says he is afraid of losing me. Although I have now switched doctors, I honestly don't know if I can trust any doctor anymore. I still want a baby so badly, but I really feel confused. What am I going to do?

An ectopic pregnancy by itself is an emotionally complex experience composed of many different losses. However, these losses are usually overshadowed by the very real threat to the woman's future fertility and the life-threatening medical emergency that accompanies most ectopic pregnancies. Friends and family often add to this process of sweeping the loss of the baby under the rug by talking only about the details of surgery.

You can trust and thank that part of you that is scared and holding you back from getting pregnant again. It knows that you are not ready to move on until you have grieved the baby you have lost. For this reason you would be better off making "an issue" out of your baby and all the other losses associated with your ectopic pregnancy. It is probably time for you to bring all your losses to the foreground so you can finally grieve for them.

The following losses are often put aside by women who have had an ectopic pregnancy. (This list is only a brief overview of these complicated issues; losses relating to identity and faith are covered more thoroughly in Chapters 1 and 8, respectively). While you may not believe all these losses are relevant to you, take the time to think about them.

- *Loss of the Baby*   The baby lost from an ectopic pregnancy is just as much a baby as any lost to miscarriage. Although the actual pregnancy was short, the plans made for this baby started long before the positive pregnancy result. The dreams you had for this child were very real and very important to you. Your baby will be missed.

- *Loss of Control*   Many patients report feeling out of control both before and after surgery. An ectopic pregnancy is usually diagnosed so late in development that the woman has to endure emergency surgery and all the accompanying trauma. Decisions about treatment are out of her control and totally in the hands of the physician, leaving her feeling powerless. After the surgery, the patient sometimes generalizes those helpless and scared feelings to other parts of her life, coming to see almost everything as being out of her control. She may even experience anxiety and feelings of panic after the surgery, especially when returning to everyday life. Before the ectopic pregnancy, she may have viewed her life as being as ordinary as the next person's, but this pregnancy loss may awaken her to the fragility of life.

- *Loss of the Image of Being Healthy*   Most of us have expectations of our bodies which we find very difficult to relinquish even if they do not match our reality. Although most infertile women are by definition as healthy as fertile women, they no longer feel healthy. Treatments, medications, doctors' visits, and surgeries all serve to make the infertile woman feel unhealthy. In addition, women who have experienced an ectopic pregnancy often lose a fallopian tube and so may feel damaged or incomplete. In addition, the remaining physical scars of the surgery are emotionally painful, constant reminders of the losses suffered.

- *Loss of Identity as a Fertile Woman*   When people lose their fertility, they lose a precious piece of themselves they never expected to lose. Women who have had their fertility compromised by an ectopic pregnancy may lose both a part of their identity (being a fertile woman) and a physical part of themselves (a fallopian tube). Because many women are told that having an ectopic pregnancy is rare (it occurs in about 1 percent of all pregnancies),[12] they begin to feel no longer part of the club of "normal" (fertile) women. This change in status is especially difficult for women, with no history of infertility prior to the ectopic pregnancy.

- *Loss of a Sense of Fairness in the World*   Unless a woman has experienced crisis before, she may be surprised at how incredibly "unfair" life suddenly seems to be after a pregnancy loss. Things about the world she once believed may no longer seem true. She may wonder why pregnancy seems so unattainable to her yet comes so easily to some women who neither want nor are equipped to parent.

- *Loss of Faith*   After an ectopic pregnancy some women experience a change in their faith. It may become stronger when they realize they survived a medical emergency. Or they may reject their beliefs, feeling God has let them down.
- *Loss of Trust in Physicians*   Even before diagnosis, ectopic pregnancies may produce physical symptoms which women report to their physicians. Many women find their concerns about these symptoms ignored. Usually the diagnosis is made only after the ectopic pregnancy becomes a medical emergency. It is understandable, then, why these women no longer trust physicians to listen to them and lose confidence in their doctor's ability to care for them in the future. Often this mistrust spreads, causing them to beware of all subsequent dealings with the medical community.
- *Loss of the Future*   Future fertility, motherhood, and family are all threatened by ectopic pregnancy. What may have been taken for granted is now uncomfortably uncertain.

Before proceeding to another pregnancy, take a good look at these losses and work on acknowledging the full range of emotions they bring up for you. Try writing about your reaction to each issue in a journal. This way you can determine whether you have truly allowed yourself to grieve. You may also want to look though the rest of this chapter and Chapter 8 for further help in working through your grief and acknowledging your loss through ritual. As you work through the losses accompanying your experience, you and your husband will be able to move toward a brighter future.

7. Does It Mean We Aren't Supposed to Be Parents?

You wait and wait to get pregnant, and the whole time you wonder, Why me? Then you finally get pregnant, and you lose the baby. By the time you get to adoption, you don't have much money or strength, but you believe it will work, so you forge ahead. That's what my wife and I did last year. We decided that independent adoption was the way to go, and we went to see a lawyer.

Within two months of our first ad we were working with a birth mother. Everything seemed to be going well. We liked her, and she liked us. Ten weeks before her due date she delivered the baby, who had many health problems. We were devastated and confused. On the one hand, we felt like he was our child and so they were our problems. On the other hand, this wasn't yet legally our baby, so we had no claim nor obligation to take him home. After struggling with this decision we ultimately decided not to adopt him. People told us we were lucky we didn't have to take a sick baby, unlike biological parents who get whatever comes their way. But we never thought of ourselves or our situation as lucky. We felt terrible and very guilty.

Again we tried to adopt, and once again we had a great relationship with the birthmother, right from the start. We talked on the phone frequently and made plans to be together for the holidays. Then we asked for a copy of her medical records and were shocked to learn she wasn't pregnant. We were so angry at everyone who had allowed this to happen—the birth mother, the lawyer, and her therapist. We didn't know where to turn.

At this point, we are not sure if we should continue to pursue adoption. Maybe we are just not supposed to be parents! We trust no one now, especially birth mothers, and can't imagine investing all this time and money only to have the same experience happen again.

Everywhere you turn, you and your wife have faced roadblocks. You have every right to be angry at a birth mother and a system that caused both of you so much pain. However, it would be unfortunate if you allowed your anger to dissuade you from becoming parents. The difficulties infertility patients face often lead them to believe they were not meant to be parents. Yet with high-tech treatments, birth control, abortion, and adoption, just about everyone in today's society can make the choice for or against becoming a parent. If you decide not to continue with adoption, know that it is because you choose not to, not because you were not supposed to.

It is understandable why you now have difficulty trusting birth mothers. It may help to see what happened to you from a different perspective. Regarding your first experience, birth defects, as sad as they are, just happen, often without any warning and through no fault of the woman carrying the child. And although your second experience deserves your wrath and mistrust, remember that it involved only *one woman,* not all birth mothers. In fact, she was not really a birth mother— just a woman who for whatever reasons decided to carry out this terrible deception. Birth mothers have the same kinds of weaknesses and strengths we all have. A "good" birth mother who chooses adoption wants what is best for the baby she is carrying; her act is selfless. Seeing birth mothers this way should help you to move forward with your adoption plans. However it is important to work through your anger and resentment toward birth mothers before you adopt. Such attitudes can have a negative impact on any children you may have in the future.

If you decide to try independent adoption again, an experienced lawyer well versed in adoption law and the acquisition of medical records up front can help you avoid this particular situation from happening again. You can obtain the name of a lawyer specializing in adoption from your local bar association. Another route to adoption is through an agency. Although most agencies have long waiting lists, the protection they afford is worth the wait for many couples. (For further discussion of adoption, see Chapter 11.)

Take the time to grieve and feel the sadness of your loss. Although a support group is the perfect setting for this, adoption loss groups are rarely offered. Therefore it may be beneficial to seek out an adoption organization or start an adoption loss group. There you will meet other couples who have had both good and bad experiences with birth mothers. Sharing your stories will help you deal with your losses.

8. Our Second Child Was Taken from Us!

Eight years ago we adopted our daughter, who is the love of our lives. For a number of reasons, mostly financial, we put off adopting a second child until six months ago. My husband, daughter, and I visited our new baby in the hospital and were allowed to feed him. The next day we took him home and introduced him to all our friends and family. I bonded right away. As hectic as that first week was, I felt happier than I have ever been.

When our baby was eight days old, the birth parents refused to sign away their rights to our son. They said they wanted to think about their decision some more. There had been no indication of any problems until that day. After that, I had a sick feeling inside of me that wouldn't go away. It was like living with a baby who was dying. Every time I looked at him, I was reminded that this might be our last day together. When the call finally came, we were instructed to deliver the baby to the birth parents the next day. That was the hardest night of our lives. We cried. I held our baby and wondered how we could let our son go. Our parents came to say goodbye to their grandson. Worst of all, my daughter had to say goodbye to her brother. Everyone I loved was dragged into this tragedy.

Our baby, who was in our home and our hearts for ten days, was being ripped out of our arms by strangers. They knew nothing about him. We could give him everything; they could give him nothing. Why were they doing this? we asked ourselves over and over.

When they took our son away, I just sat in a chair unable to move. It was as if there had been a war and everyone had died. I have never felt pain like that before.

I barely functioned for months and had no strength for anything. I went into therapy and eventually the pain lessened. My husband was devastated, but he found some relief by throwing himself into his work.

This experience has been just as devastating for our daughter. She cried more than we would have expected and remained sad for a long time. She said she wanted to tell her friends at school what had happened, but we felt it would be best if she only talked about it with her best friend and other family members, which she agreed to. She also seemed very scared whenever she saw me crying. Even though I tried to convince her I would be okay, I don't think she believed me. We want to help her get through this better, but we are not sure how. We are considering trying to adopt again. Will this help our daughter or make things worse for her?[13]

You and your entire family have suffered one of the greatest losses a parent can experience, the loss of a child. The emotional devastation left in the wake of this loss is unparalleled. There are very few differences between the way you feel and the way a biological mother feels when she has lost her child. Your feelings may be more complicated because you are mourning a child who is alive, and there are no rituals such as a funeral to help you memorialize your baby. (We discuss a memorial service for an adoption loss in Chapter 8.) Although healing from a loss of this magnitude is a slow process, you seem to be moving in the right direction and doing the best you can by getting help through a therapist. Your husband and daughter, on the other hand, sound as if they have been handling their grieving on their own. Unlike your husband, who will eventually find his own path to resolution, your daughter will need your help in dealing with this loss.

Although your daughter's crying may be especially hard to take if it brings up strong feelings for you, it also may be the best way for her to release the intense feelings she is having over the loss of her sibling. Although you feel your daughter's crying and sadness went on for too long a time and was too intense, it may have been due to the fact that she was unable to deal with her loss in her own way. Children have a wonderful innate sense about how to handle things. Too often we adults impose our own rules and standards on thought processes that operate quite differently from our own. Your daughter may have needed to talk to *her* friends about her loss, not the people you choose for her to talk with. Can you imagine your husband telling you who to talk with about your problems? By not allowing your daughter to share her story, you may also have inadvertently sent her the message that your family's loss is something to be embarrassed about or ashamed of. Lifting the ban on whom to share information with may help both of you. She may not be finished with all that she needs to say to mourn her loss. She may also benefit tremendously from knowing you trust her judgment on this matter.

In *A Silent Sorrow,* Ingrid Kohn and Perry-Lynn Moffitt describe the types of reactions children have to the loss of a sibling. Although the focus of this book is on pregnancy losses, it is logical to assume that many of the feelings overlap with those of adoption loss. The reactions that Kohn and Moffitt believe to be a part of the experience for some children include the fears and overprotectiveness you talked about. It is difficult for a child of any age to see a parent suffer; because your daughter is so young, she probably feels especially vulnerable watching you in so much pain. Do not hide how you feel; rather, assure her that you are going to be fine, but that once in a while you are very sad about the baby you lost. You can explain that everyone experiences sadness when someone or something is lost or dies, and that each person takes a different amount of time to feel better again.

She may also in some ways feel responsible for your losing the baby. Ambivalent feelings about the adoption and about some of your attention shifting away from her may have made her want the child to disappear. When the baby was taken away, she may have thought that wishing for the child to go away had made it happen.

In addition to what might be considered typical loss reactions, your daughter must also deal with the issues surrounding both your son's failed adoption and her own successful adoption. Your daughter may wonder why her brother's biological parents changed their mind and hers did not. Was she not lovable, important, or worthy enough? Such are the questions your daughter may be facing alone. Her self-esteem, no matter how intact before, may be taking a bruising on this one. She may only see that everyone is fighting for this boy and no one is fighting for her.

Keep the lines of communication as open and as clear as possible. This means being receptive to her questions and asking her questions that might help you find out what is too hard for her to tell you directly. You probably have had to learn to read between the lines with her before. Although it may be difficult for you to do this right now, it is important to try.

Trying to adopt again could make things better or worse for her. On the one hand, another failed adoption would probably leave another trail of damage that would have to be dealt with. On the other hand, a successful adoption, especially in the near future, might give her a more hopeful outlook and a sibling to share her life with.

If you do decide to go back and try to adopt again, you will surely send your daughter a strong message about what to do when life does not go as planned. You will show her how you dealt with a crisis and moved past it. She will probably grow up believing in the old adage, "If at first you don't succeed, try, try again." If that is your philosophy, then you can feel good about going ahead with your plans.

Remember that kids are very resilient and are usually able to bounce back from problems more quickly and thoroughly than adults. With your help, your daughter will be able to use this situation as a learning experience. And in the future, whenever she is faced with a loss, she will be able to show her feelings and face her sadness. Good luck to all of you. We hope that in time you will heal from this pain and resume the happiness you once found with each other.

9. How Do I Handle All These Fears?

When I was ten years old, my father died, and my mother never remarried. At twenty-one, I lost my mother to cancer. When I found my husband, I hoped we would be the family I never had. Then I had five miscarriages. After that we looked into adoption and worked with a birth mother who changed her mind right before she gave birth.

I don't think I can take this anymore. Do you know what it's like to lose everything? I thought I had dealt with all my grief, but these past few incidents have pushed me over the edge. Now I'm even scared to let my husband go out of the house; I keep thinking something will happen to him and he'll die too. Lately I've been feeling scared even when I go places. Yesterday I got so scared at the supermarket that I had to leave. I have always needed to understand the reasons behind things, but the more I try to understand what is happening to me, the more confused and angry I get. I think I'm going crazy. Can you help me make sense of this?

You have had to deal with a huge amount of loss, both recently and at a very young age. During this current time of crisis you are probably longing for the support your mother and father would have been able to provide. The good news is that you are not going crazy—there are reasons for everything you are now experiencing.

The sudden attacks of fear you are having are called panic attacks. According to David H. Barlow, Ph.D., and Michelle G. Craske, Ph.D., authors of the book *Mastery of Your Anxiety and Panic*, people who have panic attacks experience one or more of the following symptoms: "difficulty breathing, sweating, chest pain or discomfort, unsteadiness, dizziness or faintness, feelings of unreality or detachment, trembling or shaking, tingling or numbness, nausea or abdominal distress, palpitations or tachycardia, choking or smothering sensations, hot flashes or cold chills, fear of dying, fear of going crazy or losing control."[14] These authors go on to cite the statistic that "over 30% of the population has experienced some sort of panic attack during the past year, often in response to a very stressful situation. . . ."[15] While some people under high levels of stress have symptoms like migraines or ulcers, others like yourself have panic attacks. Get a medical checkup if you are experiencing these attacks, since symptoms of various medical conditions may mimic panic and they should be ruled out. If the panic symptoms persist and become problematic, you have two alternatives: drug therapy or cognitive therapy. Both have proven to be highly effective in dealing with panic. However, if your symptoms occur only occasionally and are not limiting you in any way, then it would probably be better for you to start focusing on the source of your stress.

Is it possible that you never really dealt with the past losses in your life? Try this simple exercise. Visualize a box, say a shoebox. Now visualize putting a balloon, filled to the size of a grapefruit, inside the box for each loss you have suffered in your life: your mother, your father, each of your five miscarriages and your adoption loss. Next, recognize that all major life events, whether good or bad, are highly stressful and carry some degree of loss. Put more balloons in your shoebox for all the good things such as buying a house, moving to a new area, taking a new job, and getting married. You will find that if there is too much in there, you will not be able to close the box. That is exactly what is happening to your body—too many things inside, too much pressure. When you truly work through grief, it will feel as if the balloons in the box deflate. Though they never completely disappear, they take up much less space, leaving room for the ever-changing stresses of life.

How do you deal with all this unresolved loss and subsequent stress? Look for a good grief counselor who can guide you through the process. The author of *Life Is Good-bye, Life Is Hello,* Alla Renée Bozarth, Ph.D., a priest and therapist herself, talks about her need to have another therapist help her during her own journey through loss.

> At a certain point in my last grief journey, I knew that I could not continue alone. I needed the security and protection of someone who could witness my process, as I allowed a part of myself to die. I also knew that only when we allow

ourselves to go all the way through any kind of death experience can we come out the other side into whatever life is beyond the abyss.[16]

This life beyond is one that is worth getting to, even though the road to it is never easy. Once there you will find great relief and the freedom to move ahead with your life in ways you would have never dreamed possible.

II

—

ACCEPTANCE

8

Religion, Spirituality, Myths, and Miracles
Keeping Your Faith

Of all the questions infertility patients ask themselves while they are trying to accept the reality of infertility, none is more profound than, *"Why has this happened to me?"* Day after day they search to find meaning behind this crisis. They read books, talk to other infertile couples, pray for answers, speak to the clergy, and still they come up empty, wondering what they did to deserve this. Am I so bad, so mean, so unworthy that God★ would take away my ability to have children? They ask for God's forgiveness, make deals and promise to do whatever it takes to a have a baby. No matter how good they once felt about themselves, infertility brings them to their knees, and they can only see themselves and every aspect of their lives as being "less than." A life once filled with expectations and enjoyment feels empty and chronically sad. Their relationships suffer. There seems to be no justice, and time is no longer on their side; in fact, it works against them. As the fear that this feeling will never go away mounts they begin to question whether there will ever be a light at the end of this long, dark, ugly tunnel.

For each of them the journey to the end of this crisis will be different, but where they look for answers is surprisingly similar. Some people turn to spirituality or religion to make sense of their infertility. By "spirituality" we mean the part of a person that "believes" or has "faith" no matter what the circumstances are and no matter what the current science and technology can prove to be so. Marianne Williamson, in her book *A Return to Love,* defines faith as "believing that the universe is on our side. . . . Faith is a psychological awareness of an unfolding force for good, constantly at work in all dimensions."[2]

But faith is not always easy to have, especially during the difficult times in your life. The best way to survive this period of wavering faith is to *believe in your own truth*. This means listening to that part of you that tells you what is right for you, not what is right for your parents, your spouse, your friends, or anyone else. Turn to your own beliefs and your own spirituality. For some of you this means turning

---

★ We have decided to use the term "God" to refer to a Supreme Being. Although we struggled over what gender to use when we spoke of God, we decided to go with the traditional view of God as a male, for simplification. However, we encourage you to use your own choice for gender and name for the Absolute, such as God, Goddess, the Almighty, and so on.[1]

to God or religion, in whatever form it takes. For others, it will mean going deep inside yourself to a place of inner peace and meaning, and still others turn to rituals or spiritual objects.

Whatever shape or form your own truth takes, recognize that it will not always feel comfortable. After all, infertility has hit you like a bolt of lightening. Your body is not working the way it should, your dreams and hopes for the future are at stake, and your emotions are intense. You may feel very angry, especially at God. These are typical but unsettling reactions for many people. Allow yourself to have your feelings. Faith is not about believing that you will get what you want, when you want it, the way you want it. Rather, it is about trusting you can reach your goals, as long as you do not insist that there is only one means to an end. As one woman who eventually became a parent stated, "If it wasn't for my infertility we would not have been blessed with our children. I thank God every day for bringing them to us."

Such sentiments were echoed by those religious and spiritual leaders we interviewed for this chapter, among them were a Catholic priest, a Unitarian minister, a Presbyterian minister, a Reform rabbi, a minister at an African American Methodist Episcopalian Church, a pastor at a large conservative Christian church, and a shamanic healer. Each shared their view of infertility with us and discussed ways in which their congregation could express and come to terms with their pain and anger toward God and yet in the end receive the gift of faith. In each of the questions in this chapter, we incorporated this spectrum of beliefs to give our readers a wider perspective on the religious interpretations of infertility. We also discuss the various ways infertile individuals can find their way back to their faith and in the process find a new and stronger spirituality.

We encourage you to begin your own healing path. While you are directing yourself toward resolving your infertility, try not to drain the energy away from your emotional and spiritual self. As Joan Borysenko says in *Fire in the Soul,*

> At no time are we more conscious of the darkness than in the midst of a dark night of the soul. And at no other time are we less conscious of the light, although it has never abandoned us. In its concealment it forces us to stand on the threshold and commit ourselves to becoming new. If we can trust and believe that our dark night has come in service of the light, then we can breathe through the transition and do the work that is necessary to prepare for the birth.[3]

QUESTIONS TO ASK YOURSELF ABOUT INFERTILITY AND SPIRITUALITY

Below are some questions to ask yourself. Write your answers down in a journal (see Appendix I for a discussion of the techniques of journaling). This will allow you to review them later to see how your faith and spirituality have changed over the course of your infertility.

1. How has the crisis of infertility affected your relationship with God?
2. How has infertility changed your view of the meaning of life?
3. How has infertility changed your view of human nature?
4. How has infertility confirmed or changed any of your previous spiritual or moral beliefs?
5. How has infertility changed your views of right or wrong, of sin or injustice?
6. What have you learned thus far about the personal meaning of the crisis? Do you view it as a punishment of sorts? As a purely random event you just happen to find yourself in, which has little to do with your personality or morality? Or some other way?[4]

1. Can My Faith Be Restored?

In my family I was the "good daughter" according to my parents: I did almost everything my parents wanted me to do. My parents were very religious, so we all went to church on Sunday, attended Bible classes every week, and said our prayers every night. Although my faith was never as strong as my parents', I felt compelled to go along with what they believed was right.

I met my husband my first year of Bible college. The following year we had a big church wedding. We both felt truly blessed to have found each other. We became very involved in church activities because we love children so much: we both taught Sunday school, and my husband led the youth group. We couldn't wait to start our own family. That was four years ago. Since then, we have endured every test and treatment for infertility currently available, and nothing has worked.

I wake up every morning wondering who this God is that we believe in so strongly. My parents said He would always be there for me. Where is He now that I need Him? I've stopped praying to God for His help. It just makes me mad when He doesn't respond. I want desperately to have faith again. Can I get it back?

Many people's beliefs about God carry over from childhood to adulthood with few revisions. Often it is not until they are faced with a challenge or crisis that they reevaluate these beliefs. You have been given such a challenge through infertility. Whether you get your "faith" back depends mainly on your ability to grow spiritually.

The first thing you might want to do is question what your parents meant when they said God would always be there for you. Did you, like many people, believe He was there to answer your prayers, grant wishes, or to keep you happy? Or did they mean that *God would be there on your darkest days, to hear your prayers, and accept your anger until you were over this crisis in your life?* As Lynda Rutledge Stephenson says in her book *Give Us a Child,* "I can't believe that God stayed up one night and decided that we'd never have a child of our own. Instead, I believe that the laws of nature were set in motion and very very rarely have they ever been preempted [by God], and I am not presumptuous enough to demand such attention." To be spiritually healthy, you have to make the leap from using prayer to get what you want, to using it to become closer to God and to let Him be close to you.[5]

Getting past your disappointment and anger toward God in order to get closer to Him is not easy, but, according to the religious leaders we spoke with, the best way do this is to *accept the fact that you are angry.* This can be a difficult task for those who grew up believing that such anger was blasphemous and could cause God in His ire to retaliate in some way. Letting God know how angry and upset you are is an acceptable, understandable, part of the letting-go process that must take place in order for you to make peace with your spirituality.

Think about the times you have been so angry at a friend that you decided to not talk to her anymore. You might have just cut yourself off from her and went on with your life as if nothing had ever happened. But maybe her absence began to plague you, so you called to see if there was any room for reconciliation. After speaking to her you may have realized that it did not matter that you were not able to work out all your problems. You still wanted her in your life. It is the same way with your infertility and God. Unlike humans, who may turn away from anger, your faith can be a source toward which you can safely direct your most intense feelings.

Stephenson describes how her faith works for her:

> Choosing to stay open to my faith doesn't mean I do not still want a child, or that I give up. And it doesn't mean I'll not have relapses into my own little personal hells of peer-pressure, of self-pity, of slamming doors and shaking fists. But, if this works out the way I think it will, I'll be relapsing less and less, and finding my faith more and more—on the same level that Job did. Not finding answers so much as "presence." And if so, I'll remember that this isn't all there is,

that life isn't for having, doing and wanting. And on the days that I do, I'll find that God is God, and that He loves me—Being to being. And I'll find that such belief is sufficient. For the moment. For the day. For the future, children or no.[6]

2. How Can Prayer Help Me?

After three years of infertility, I finally got pregnant. Needless to say, my husband and I were unbelievably happy. But that feeling was short-lived. I miscarried in my third month. I'll never forget that horrible day, when the bleeding started. That same evening I had a D&C. I came home from the hospital the next morning and just lay in bed all day crying. For the next few days my feelings were so overwhelming I thought I would die.

A few weeks have passed since then, and I have been trying to make some sense out of all of this. My mother encouraged me to talk to our priest. He's known me since I was a child—he even married me and my husband—but I wasn't sure if he was the right person to talk to. I went to see him anyway. Although he was very supportive, the only real advice he gave me was to pray to God. Why will this help?

Priests have seen many people receive solace by turning to prayer during their most difficult times. Recognizing your pain, your priest was no doubt trying to share this knowledge with you. Exactly how prayer works, however, is a mystery that humans may never unravel, but there is mounting evidence that prayer can be helpful to people in many ways.

For some people prayer offers a sense of peace and comfort away from the hectic nature of human existence, especially in our fast-paced society. For those who believe in the concept of "the divine within," prayer can put them in touch with an element or quality of the Supreme Being. Still others, like Larry Dossey, physician and cochairman of the Panel on Mind/Body Interventions, at the Office of Alternative Medicine, National Institutes of Health, believes that prayer has healing and restorative capabilities.

In his book *Healing Words*, Dossey cites many studies in which scientists have sought evidence for prayers' power. The results are impressive. In one study,

a computer assigned 393 patients admitted to the coronary care unit at San Francisco General Hospital to either a group that was prayed for by home prayer groups or to a group . . . that was not remembered in prayer. . . . The prayed for patients were five times less likely than the unremembered group to require antibiotics . . . [and] three times less likely to develop pulmonary edema. . . ."[7]

While these findings are significant, no studies have been done on the relationship between prayer and infertility. Therefore, we could not even begin to presume how praying could specifically impact your chances of carrying a baby. Prayer is highly personal. For some it is a way to heal and helps them get through the pain and crisis of infertility.

If you decide you want to use prayer as a healing method, here are some prayers we found inspiring. The first is "The Serenity Prayer," part of a longer poem by Reinhold Niebuhr, and used by many 12-Step programs:

> O God grant me
> the *serenity* to accept the things I cannot change,
> the *courage* to change the things I can, and
> the *wisdom* to know the difference.[8]

Another prayer we found comforting is from Psalm 139:

> Where can I go from your Spirit?
> Where can I flee from your presence?
> If I go up to the heavens, you are there;
> if I make my bed in the depths, you are there;
>
> If I rise on the wings of the dawn,
> if I settle on the far side of the sea,
> even there your hand will guide me,
> your right hand will hold me fast.

We hope that you will find a peaceful way to the resolution that is right for you.

3. How Does the Jewish Religion Treat Adoption?*

After five years of experiencing infertility and all the craziness that goes along with it, my husband and I finally got to the point where we wanted to adopt a baby. Since we have a very close knit Jewish family, we wanted to tell everyone our ex-

---

* Much of the information in this answer can be found in Michael Gold's book *And Hanna Wept: Infertility, Adoption and the Jewish Couple* (Jewish Publication Society, Philadelphia, 1988).

citing news. My family was very happy, but my husband's family was upset. They want our family to maintain our Judaic roots and are concerned about the religion of the child we adopt. They say if we adopt a child whose mother isn't Jewish, he or she won't be a real Jew. Are they right about this? It's hard enough to find any birth mother, but what are the chances of finding a Jewish one?

The reaction of your in-laws must have been difficult to witness considering how much you had invested in your decision. You could share with them the fact that although Jews put more emphasis on bloodlines than most religions, adoption is viewed as a *mitzvah,* a great blessing. You could also remind your in-laws that many stories in the Bible—those of Sarah, Rachel, Esther, and Moses—provide evidence that Jews have been open to adoption since the beginning of time.

The issue of whether a child should only be adopted from a Jewish birth mother is confusing because the answer varies according to whom you talk to. For some rabbis the adoption of a Jewish child is preferable to a non-Jewish one, while for others the match is less important. It depends on how the rabbi interprets Jewish law. Most Jews today, however, adopt children who are not Jewish by birth and choose to convert them. These babies can be of Caucasian as well as nonwhite descent. It makes absolutely no difference in the eyes of Jewish law whether the baby has similar skin tones to its adoptive parents; the only essential is that the child be converted in the manner ordained by Jewish law.

For Jews of Orthodox and Conservative faiths, this law requires a male infant to go through a ceremony called a *bris* or *brit milah,* during which a Mohel (a person ordained by the synagogue) performs a circumcision and says a special conversion blessing. Even if the baby was circumcised before, the ceremony has to be repeated in a religious fashion with a symbolic circumcision taking place. Both female and male children are required to go through a *mikvah,* a ritual in which the child is immersed in a natural body of water. Three rabbis, referred to as a tribunal,★ are present at the ceremony and provide the appropriate blessings. Reform and Reconstructionist congregants may choose instead to have their children named in the synagogue. For these two groups this naming ceremony along with the commitment to give the child a Jewish education legitimize the conversion.

The conversion of a child is a profound and happy occasion. Families typically

---

★ Some people, regardless of their affiliation (Reform, Conservative, etc.), feel more comfortable with a Rabbinical tribunal performing the *mikvah.* They feel there will be fewer questions in the future as to the legitimacy of the conversion.

have a party following a conversion to celebrate the "symbolic birth of the adopted child into the Jewish community."[10]

Once the child is formally converted, he or she is pronounced a Jew and is encouraged to go through the traditional ceremony of a *bar mitzvah* or *bat mitzvah,* at the age of majority (thirteen plus one day for a boy and twelve plus one day for a girl). Although the *bar* or *bat mitzvah* is not mandatory, it is typically the time when a converted child publicly declares the desire to continue as a Jew throughout adult life. At this point the child is given the opportunity to reaffirm his or her faith in Judaism.

Despite the Jewish community's acceptance of an adopted child, the question remains as to whether your in-laws can emotionally accept an adopted grandchild. In his book *And Hanna Wept,* Michael Gold states that

> sometimes grandparents and other family members are reluctant to accept an adopted child into the family. This is particularly true of European-born grandparents, who are often more old fashioned about the proper way to build a family. Such grandparents need to be educated about the importance of adoption in Jewish history. Ideally time and love will win them over.[11]

Most grandparents tell us that although they were hesitant at first, they now feel blessed by grandchildren now part of their family. They take great pleasure in seeing how happy their children are to be parents and no longer think about the fact that their grandchildren were Gentile, when they first arrived.

We suggest that you talk to your Rabbi about your desire to adopt and find out if there are other adoptive parents in the congregation that can speak to you. It might also be possible to bring your in laws with you when you talk to the Rabbi and with the other adoptive parents. Include them in as much as possible. Most likely, all they need is some reassurance that things will work out. And they usually do, we see it happen all the time.

4. How Does "Be Fruitful and Multiply" Apply to Me?

"Be fruitful and multiply," one of the first verses in Genesis*—it haunts me every time I go to church. I sit there every week trying to figure out the relevance

---

* "Be fruitful and multiply. Fill the earth and master it and rule the fish of the sea, the birds of the sky, and all the living things that creep on earth," Genesis 1:28.

of this verse to a person who can't bear children. Now my husband and I are strongly considering living without children, but I cannot help but wonder what God will think of us. Will we still be recognized by God and our Church as a family?

The religious leaders we interviewed offered us their view of Genesis 1:28 with regard to infertile couples. Each of them, from the most conservative to the most liberal, believed that those who did not or could not fulfill the literal interpretation of the mandate to be fruitful and multiply could find other ways of directing the same nurturing energy and meaning in their lives. They all agreed that couples could give life and love to something other than a child. They also shared the belief that a couple choosing to live child-free after struggling with infertility would not be viewed by God or the religious community as inferior or "sinful."

Consider talking to your own minister, who might help you find inner peace and a place that is comfortable for you and your husband within your spiritual community.

In the turmoil of trying to get pregnant, it is easy to forget that life is not just about making babies; it is also about giving something back to the world that is morally and spiritually precious. To do this you need to acknowledge that you *are* a family—a family of two—and that your contributions to the world, whatever they may be, are just as important as the contributions made by families with children.

5. Holiday Services Are Painful for Me

People in pain often come to church for solace, but since my struggles with infertility began, going to church has, on a number of occasions, caused me even more hurt. One service in particular was extremely difficult to get through. The kids in Sunday school had decided to do something special for Mother's Day, so they handed out flowers to all the mothers. As they gave my mother and all my sisters their hyacinth, I sat there fighting back the tears. I kept thinking, What about me? What if I never become a mother? I am so tired of feeling like an outcast. Doesn't the church realize that there are infertile women who would give anything to be mothers and receive those flowers?

It is common for us to hear from women and men struggling with infertility that their house of worship is no longer the sanctuary it once was, especially on certain holidays. We asked the clergy we interviewed whether they were aware of couples in their congregation experiencing infertility, and their answer was a resounding *no!* Although they were familiar with infertility and most counseled a few couples who were trying to make some decisions about it, they were unaware of how common the problem is. They were also unaware that the sermons or prayers mentioned on holidays like Mother's Day might alienate infertile couples from their church or synagogue.

All the clergy we spoke with promised to acknowledge the feelings and needs of infertile couples during future services. The best way to help your church meet your needs and those of the other infertile couples in the congregation is for you and others like you to educate your priest or minister about infertility. This can be done through a letter, a phone call, or a private conversation. You can also suggest certain readings about infertility that you have found helpful. Decide on the method you are most comfortable with, and make the commitment to inform your minister about your suffering. You will probably find, as we did in our interviews, that he or she will be open to exploring and addressing your needs and may even be willing to plan a service or public reflection on the topic of infertility.

6. Our Church Says No to Our Infertility Treatments

My wife and I were raised Catholic. We have always observed our religion's practices and participated in services as well as the activities of the church. The church and our faith have always been there throughout our infertility. Recently, however, our lives and our faith have come to an impasse we can't seem to resolve.

Our doctor has recommended that we try inseminations as the next step in our infertility treatment. If that doesn't work, he has suggested we consider using donor sperm. I know that the Pope's encyclical strictly prohibits the use of donor sperm, but we still plan on trying it if necessary. This will not be easy, however. We are not sure how our family and our priest will react to us. We doubt they are going to be very understanding. How have other couples handled this decision?

We understand your dilemma of wanting to have children desperately yet remain loyal to your faith and family. "Couples with strong faith and moral lives run the risk of suffering more intensely than couples with less religiously influenced outlooks. . . ."[12] Let's first see why that is, and then we will discuss some options you and your wife can consider.

Arthur Griel, in his book *Not Yet Pregnant,* says that pregnancy was once viewed as something that "just happened" between two people—the mechanics were somewhat of a mystery. Today the mystery has been removed, and we tend to view fertility as a biological function that we can master. This is where the paradox begins for couples like yourselves who have grown up with the religious view that conception is a miracle and should be left in the hands of God. This explanation is most likely not as convincing as it once was for you because infertility appears not as an "unexplainable disability to be accepted but as a technical problem to be overcome." To accept the "God's will" philosophy implies a spirit of resignation which "does not currently exist in the pursuit of infertility treatment."[13]

Although the Catholic religion has remained firm in its position on the use of donor sperm, many couples come to decisions that have gone against the Church's doctrine. They justify their resolution by interpreting the Church's policies as antiquated, and view the use of donor sperm as a kind of technological adoption. They also see the Catholic Church's pressure to have children and its denial of certain infertility treatments as sending a mixed message. Elizabeth Noble, in her book *Having Your Baby by Donor Insemination,* says that "although donor insemination disassociates procreation from conjugal love, the relationship continues for the couple, and the arrangement for the genetic component of their child is done of their consensual free choice, and can be seen as part of the love the couple expresses for each other."[14]

Many Catholics that have gone against a policy dictated by the Pope still maintain their affiliation with the Church. The priest we spoke with said that some priests believe infertile couples must follow their conscience and do whatever they feel necessary to create a family. As one priest stated in the journal *U.S. Catholic,* "It is important to distinguish between infallible and fallible Church teachings. It is very blessed to belong to the teaching Church and to have the guidance for life but we should not condemn persons who have carefully formed their consciences, even if their consciences are contrary to fallible teaching."[15] It also interesting to note that a number of Catholic countries, including Spain, France, and Italy, have donor insemination programs.

For some Catholic couples one of the most important by-products of their decision to conceive through a donor was the creation of a strong belief system. Both spouses had to believe that what they were doing was right and morally correct, especially if they chose to disclose how their child was conceived. Vern Smith, a family practitioner and an infertility patient, tells couples to "Make sure you understand everything that is going on or could go on. Be sure to deal with every little speed bump that you come across as a couple. Don't say, I'll chalk this one up for me, this one for you. Make sure [you understand] how each of you feels about each item and try not to give just yes or no answers to each other."[16]

Be sure you talk with your wife about the effects your families' reactions might have on you as a couple and eventually as parents. Fortunately for most couples, when families see how happy their children are to be parents, the genetic background of the child almost always becomes less and less important. Your other option is not to tell family members of your child's origins. Before making this decision, we encourage you to consider how you would feel carrying this information with you for the rest of your child's life. (For further discussion on the impact of the decision to use donor sperm, see Chapter 11.)

7. My Infertility Feels Like a Punishment

I can't figure out what I've done to deserve infertility. I feel like God is punishing me. I may not be perfect, but I've never done anything *that* bad. I have friends who've cheated on their taxes and others who've had affairs while they were married, and they've all gotten pregnant with no problem. I've tried to be a better person and I even started going to mass regularly, but nothing seems to help.

This is probably your first encounter with the harsh reality that bad things happen to all of us whether we are "good" or "bad." Because it is so hard to accept that we have no control over these difficulties, there is a natural tendency to look for a guilty party, someone to point the finger at, such as a physician, a parent, a spouse, or, all too often, ourselves.

Griel cites Melvin Lerner, a social psychologist, who asserts that "people need to believe in a just world in which people are punished for misdeeds and rewarded for proper behavior. [Lerner] contends that some people in situations like infertility will hold themselves responsible for their condition."[17] Since most of us were raised to believe that if we are "good," we would get what we wanted from life, this explanation is understandable. Many infertile couples make bargains with themselves and with God. Some people think that if they become more involved in their religion, God might answer their prayers. However, is the return to religious roots motivated by a sense of desperation and fear rather than a desire to get support and comfort from God?

We all need the reassurance that God does not punish us when we do something wrong. If He did, we would all live in a state of purgatory. As one rabbi said, "I don't believe that I have to wear thick glasses because I sneaked a look at Playboy when I was a teenager." He believes that finding a more honest way back to

God comes from the need to see God as forgiving and comforting, rather than judgmental and disciplinary.

The most reassuring response we can give you is to emphasize that *you* did not cause your infertility. You did not do anything in your past that you are being punished for, and God is not trying to send you a message that you are undeserving. Infertility attacks people randomly, just like cancer, diabetes, or car accidents. Go easy on yourself. Remember that you are simply a human being whose body is not functioning correctly. Your job now is to focus on improving your reproductive system to increase your probability of conceiving and reducing your stress level as much as possible. (See Appendix I for ways to deal with stress.) You need to be good to yourself and treat your mind, body, and spirit as best you can during this difficult time.

8. What about Crystals, Fertility Charms, Myths, and Miracles?

I have been trying to get pregnant for the past five years. Throughout my treatment, I've tried to increase our luck by using crystals to give me positive energy, but so far it hasn't worked. Other people have suggested that I put fertility symbols around my house, drink raspberry and other herbal teas, and even make love on red sheets. Before I invest any money or hope in these remedies, I'd like to know whether you know of any other fertility "charms" that have worked for patients?

The use of "fertility charms" has risen lately due to the fact that more and more people are involving themselves in New Age philosophies and practices. Many infertility patients, understandably desperate to find a cure and faced with a never-ending stream of tests and treatments, are increasingly willing to try anything that sounds promising and noninvasive.

The need to "cure" infertility has been in existence since time immemorial. Women currently using crystals or drinking herbal remedies are carrying on a tradition that began centuries before them. For instance, in Scotland there was a rock way out in the River Dee with a hole large enough for a person to fit through. It was once believed that a woman could overcome her fertility problems by swimming out to the rock and passing herself through the hole.[18]

Native Americans believed the earth had the power to heal an infertile person. A Yuma tale tells of a couple who requested the help of a medicine man. First, he diagnosed which partner was having the infertility problem by having them both lie on the ground and then lifting each of them up under the arms. When he determined that it was the female who was "lacking seed," he thrust his right arm into the soil and covered her with the course sand he had retrieved. At the same time he blew smoke on her belly, which according to the legend, made her pregnant.[19]

Of course, these stories are about ancient beliefs that included cures that today we would consider miraculous. But, as Stephenson says in *Give Us a Child,*

> miracles, however they happen and whoever they happen to, are exceptions not rules. That's the nature of miracles. To make them something we can earn with the right poundage of faith is to belittle the wondrous, to have control over the supernatural. And in effect, if we were able to do this, if we could make miracles the rule, we'd have to redefine what a miracle is, because it wouldn't be a miracle anymore.[20]

Therefore, if the reality is that a miracle cure will most likely not be found for infertility, then is there any validity to all the hype about holding crystals, drinking herbal teas, lighting candles, and burning incense while making love on red satin sheets? According to Irene Siegel, a holistic psychotherapist and healer from Long Island, New York, these methods are not miracle cures but tools one can use during the healing process.[21]

Currently used in technology to increase energy flow, crystals are also believed to be helpful in channeling positive cosmic energy to the individual. Quartz is the most common crystal used, although there are other kinds of gems recommended for varying ailments. Siegel emphasizes, however, that it is not a power inherent in the crystal itself that heals but rather the *intention behind its use.* Therefore, the person holding the crystal must be clear about what she or he wants from the crystal's energy. Crystals can be used as amplifiers to enhance the healing process and "cleanse an emotional or physical block" that could be a factor in infertility. A person can "program" the crystal to do this by calling on or pulling in energy from a higher frequency to aid in the unblocking. The frequency of the energy being pulled in is believed to be higher than the energy causing the block and can therefore override the problem and open the obstruction.

Siegel believes, as do other spiritual healers, that a malfunction in the body indicates an imbalance that is not only physical but emotional and spiritual as well. Using crystals, drinking herbal remedies, or participating in meditation and visualization, and so forth can be means for infertility patients to get in touch with parts of themselves they may be unaware of, that are possibly even divine-like. In this way they may be able to restore inner balance and find a sense of peace within themselves. As Louise L. Hay says in *Heart Thoughts,* "In order to reprogram the subconscious mind, you need to relax the body. Release the tension. Let the emotions go. Get to a state of openness and receptivity. You are always in charge. You are always safe." Once patients can achieve this, they can regain their spiritual side and come to terms with whatever the outcome is of their infertility. "A tragedy can turn out to be our greatest good, if we approach it in ways we can grow."[22]

If you feel open enough to consider these alternative healing methods, then by all means get as much information as you can about the best way to use them. Appendix II lists some of the organizations that can help you. We have also provided some meditation and visualization techniques in Appendix I.

9. We'd Like a Service for Our Miscarriage

After six years of infertility, I finally got pregnant. But, it was short-lived. I lost the baby at sixteen weeks. Needless to say, we were devastated. Our friends encouraged us to have a memorial service for the baby, but we had never heard of such a ceremony. Since we are new to the area and not affiliated with any one church, we are unsure of where to turn.

Your concern for the well-being of your baby's soul or spirit is a common issue for bereaved parents. As Ingrid Kohn and Perry-Lynn Moffitt emphasize in *A Silent Sorrow*, "No matter when your loss occurred in the pregnancy, you deserve the comfort of knowing that your God has not forsaken you and that your baby has not gone from this world unnoticed or unblessed."[23]

Since you are unsure of where to turn, try contacting the hospital for the telephone numbers of their visiting clergy. Once you locate someone, you can discuss your feelings and ask that either a prayer be said during services at the clergyperson's church or a special memorial service be conducted for your baby. It is important that you follow your heart when you decide what kind of service you would like. (See the answer to the next question for ideas.) We wish you peace in your search for comfort.

10. Is There a Goodbye Service for an Adoption Loss?

My husband and I have been trying to adopt a baby for the past year. Two months ago, we got a call from a birth mother who said her baby was due in a few days. When we got the call that the baby had been born, we were so ecstatic, we could have flown to the state she lived in without the aid of a plane! Our prayers were finally going to be answered. Everything went smoothly. The birth mother signed all the papers in the hospital, and the very next day we brought our daughter home. It was just as I had always dreamed: the house was filled with my family and friends, and everywhere there were pink balloons that said, "It's a girl!" What a relief, after all those years.

Three days later we got a call from our lawyer telling us the birth mother had changed her mind and wanted "her baby" back. What followed were the worst weeks of my life. I thought all the losses we had endured during our infertility were hard, but nothing held a candle to the intensity of the grief we now felt.

We were grateful for the support we received from our families and friends. Two friends of ours who had lost children of their own—one through miscarriage and the other a stillbirth—were especially helpful to us. They seemed to know exactly what we were going through and what we needed to hear. We realized from talking to these people that a major difference in our experience was that we never said goodbye to our daughter in a religious service. Is there any religion that would honor our request to perform a service for the daughter we lost?

Your description of your loss reminds us of the words of Vernell Klassen Miller, who writes in *Meditations for Adoptive Parents*:

> Our loss was nonetheless a death; a life was taken from us finally as death takes a life. . . . After all, we did have a child, if only briefly, and the means by which we bore that child made no difference in our feelings. . . . [We] found that the assumption we [had] shared with so many people—that adoption was second best—had vanished. We knew better—if only by the measure of our grief.[24]

You were very lucky to have had wonderfully supportive people around you during such a devastating time in your life. Their recognition that the loss you suffered was the same as their biological losses is an enlightened view more and more people are just now coming to. Society has been very slow to recognize these painful losses. If not for the Jessica DeBoer case in the summer of 1993, the devastation of adoption loss would probably still be unacknowledged. It is this lack of recognition that is most likely responsible for the fact that there are no established rituals that attend to the grief of the adoptive parents who have suffered such a loss. It will be up to you and your husband to establish your own ritual to acknowledge the loss of your daughter. Even though you may find it difficult to imagine others seeing how grieved you are over the loss of your child, a "public ritual" with loved ones can provide the catharsis that begins a healthy grieving process.[25]

Marilyn Black Phemister's poem "Tears in Season" speaks to the importance of rituals and loss:

I was down—
all the way
below the bottom.

I don't know how
I got up.
I remember weeping
a long time—
until someone
wept with me.

Then
my weeping stopped.[26]

If you decide to create your own ritual, you can enlist the help of others such as family members, friends, or clergy. Involving these people may make the task of creating a meaningful service less daunting. The following suggestions for creating your own goodbye service were proposed by Kohn and Moffitt, the authors of *A Silent Sorrow.* Since the mourning rituals in that book focus directly on pregnancy loss and stillbirth, we have adapted their guidelines here for adoption loss.

GOODBYE SERVICE[27]

- Pay close attention to what you want the ceremony to accomplish as well as who you would like to have present.
- Just like biological parents, you too fantasized what the future would hold for your daughter and for you as her parents. Share those dreams at the goodbye service.
- If you named the baby, we suggest you refer to her by her adoptive name during the service.* Her birth parents will probably call her by another name, but that is not your concern. What is important is that she be recognized by you and the people close to you as your daughter.
- Ask those close to you to contribute their feelings about your daughter at the ceremony. This can be a source of comfort for you and instill a sense of community among them.
- Incorporate prayers into the service that are appropriate for the situation. Your clergyperson will be helpful in choosing some, or you can write your own.

---

* In cases of adoption loss where the parents have not seen or held the child, it is advisable to give the child a name in order for the grieving process to have focus.

• Designing a memory book of your daughter including pictures, clothing, locks of hair, legal papers, and so on will be a source of memories for you and can be present during the service so others can see and understand how much a part of your life she was.

Whatever you include in your ceremony to help you say goodbye to your daughter, it will be special and meaningful because it is coming from your heart.

9

Decision Making and Infertility . . .
Moving On

When one door of happiness closes, another opens. But often we look so long at the closed door that we do not see the one that has opened for us. We must find all the open doors, and if we believe in ourselves we will find them and make ourselves and our lives as beautiful as God intended.

—Attributed to Helen Keller[1]

This chapter is about making tough decisions. But it is also about creating new dreams, moving forward, and seeing that there are many ways to create a family. It is about the beginning of resolution.

The decision to end medical treatment is a difficult choice that requires a good solid look inside yourself to face some tough questions. It is a process that couples come to gradually, sometimes with conviction, other times slipping back for a brief time into medical treatment and then eventually letting go.

Take a look at the accompanying diagram. The infertility journey is composed of various options: medical intervention, adoption, child-free living,

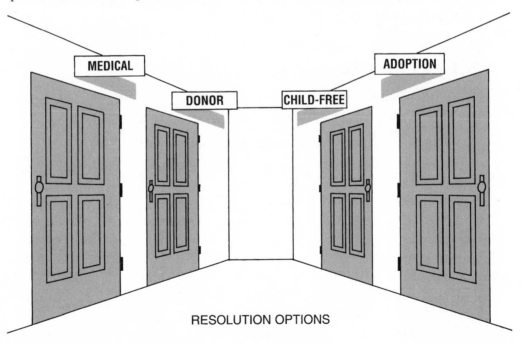

RESOLUTION OPTIONS

and third-party reproduction such as donor surrogacy and embryo adoption.

The journey begins at the door marked "medical." Most who pass through it believe the answer to their problems will be solved by medical intervention. The physician's office becomes a safe place where doctors, staff, drugs, and procedures promise the goal of biological parenthood.

For many infertile couples, hope eventually fades into disappointment as medical procedures fail to produce a child. The pursuit of fertility is a long and exhausting process that takes too much away from the individual and the couple. They feel robbed of happiness, of self-control, and of everything they had in their lives before the struggle with infertility began. As Lynda Rutledge Stephenson says,

> There will come a moment in this crisis when your own realistic side will pop through with that question, What if never? . . . But for everyone who doesn't have a successful pregnancy, the moment will come. It is a moment that you *allow* yourself to think of Plan B, about the possibility, about the options, the choices, about redefining life as you want it to be."[2]

Once the couple confronts the "what if never" question, they close the medical door a bit and begin taking small, slow steps to explore other options. They assess how they feel and imagine what it would be like to create their family through adoption, child-free living, or third-party reproduction. They begin to see that in order to close the medical door completely, they must let go of their original dream and replace it with another.

Where are you in the process now? Which doors are open and which are closed? Knowing where you are can be the first step in moving ahead.

How do you make the decision to move to the next door? You need to consider both the rational and the emotional side of continuing your medical treatment. As John D. Arnold says in his book *Make Up Your Mind,* any major life decision requires exploration of both the logical and emotional.[3]

The logical/rational side has to assess how much more you can take of medical treatment—financially, physically, and careerwise. You will want to look at the toll your infertility is taking on your relationships with your spouse, your friends, and your family. Finally, you need to decide how many more treatments and drugs your body will be able to handle.

The emotional piece of the decision is not as easy to understand because it involves feelings that concern your identity. These feelings become challenged when we experience infertility because we have failed to meet not only the expectations we have of ourselves but the expectations we believe our family, friends, and society have for us. (See Chapter 1 for a full discussion of the issue.)

So, in evaluating whether you are ready to end medical treatment, you have to look at exactly what your fertility means to you. One of the best ways to help you analyze these feelings is to separate how you feel about reproduction from your feelings about nurturing. Traditionally, most couples have seen reproduction and nurturing as one unit, as if they cannot have one without the other. However, as they go through infertility, they discover that reproduction and nurturing do not have to go hand in hand. Look at the accompanying diagram. What weighs more for you, the desire to nurture or the desire to reproduce?

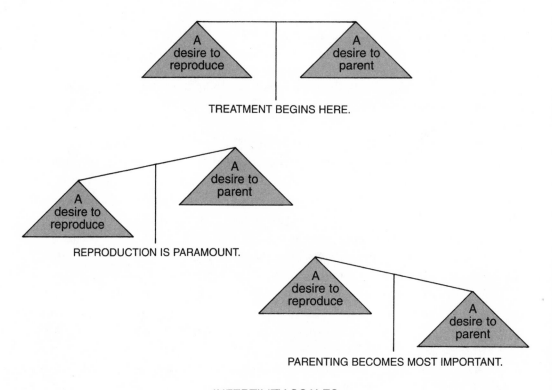

INFERTILITY SCALES

The scale will usually tip to one side or the other depending on where you are in the treatment process. When first entering medical treatment, the scale is fairly balanced. As time marches on and the desire for pregnancy becomes all-consuming, the scale tips in the reproduction direction. Later on, as the process becomes exhausting, your path to resolution can take one of two directions. You may find that the real issue is being a parent, that where the baby comes from matters less and less; at this point the scale tips to the nurturing side, and you may start looking into adoption as a way to create your family. Or you find that the genetic origin of a child remains the paramount issue, so you might choose child-free living as your path to resolution.

When and if you decide to leave medical treatment, there will be things you will be giving up, no matter which way the scales are tipped. And along with these losses will come pain and sadness. This grief is a normal and healthy part of letting go, even though our culture, especially when it comes to reproductive losses, prefers not to acknowledge it. If you do not run away from these feelings, you will be able to move ahead with a clean slate, unencumbered by old, stored-up pain.

In this chapter you will find questions about what to do if your partner has different feelings about ending treatment, what to do when finances run out, how to decide if it's too soon to end medical treatment, and how to deal with lack of communication between you and your spouse during this turning point in the infertility experience. Our answers are not meant to be an exact map for you to follow but rather guidelines to lead you through your own decision-making process.

We know from our own personal and professional experiences that ending medical treatment, although difficult and sad, is truly liberating. It marks an ending but also a beginning—a renewal of hope and possibility. As Alexandra Stoddard explained so beautifully to us and in her book *Making Choices,* "The ability to make choices can be life transforming. Nothing is preordained or predestined. It is our personal responsibility to choose for ourselves and live with our decisions. Simply doing so is a step toward freedom."[4] And giving yourself the freedom to choose is giving yourself a future.

1. What Exactly Is Resolution?

My wife and I are at the point where we would like to stop pursuing medical treatment and begin looking into adoption. Everything we've read about adoption says that you must "resolve" your infertility before moving on to adoption. What are they talking about? Isn't the decision to stop medical treatment resolution?

Resolution of infertility is a slow process and occurs in stages. The decision to stop medical treatment and consider adoption marks only the beginning of resolution, not the final stage. Another involves letting go: grieving the loss of reproduction and of nurturing a biological child. The final stage of resolution begins after you have become a parent through some nonbiological means (such as adoption or surrogacy) or after living child-free for a period of time. Most people find that true resolution comes when their family is complete and when the memories of the infertility experience begin to fade into the background. They once again rejoin the world. A new reality exists for them, different from their original dream but equally as wonderful. They also come to understand that even though they have moved on, their feelings about infertility have not vanished. Going to a baby shower or seeing a pregnant relative might bring back these feelings, but not nearly as intensely as when they were involved in treatment. (For further discussion of this stage, see the Epilogue.)

Since you have decided to end medical treatment, it would be beneficial to examine your feelings of loss. Grief is such a dreaded emotion in our society that many people seek to deny it. In order to grieve, you must first acknowledge that the grief exists. Ask yourself and your spouse if you have let go of the parts of you that wanted so desperately to reproduce. (See Chapter 1 for an in-depth discussion of the effects of infertility on identity.) Spend some time going down memory lane. Look at all the events that led up to your decision to adopt. Remember the failed cycles and the monthly ups and downs. Remember how it was when there was hope that a treatment or drug would work. What was it like when the hope began to fade? Did you say goodbye to the dreams and the children that would have been created from those cycles?

Dealing with these memories can be hard and may bring up lonely and sad feelings. In the final letting-go stage, you need to find comfort from others and make your losses as real as possible by ritualizing them. Funerals and other ceremonies serve the role of validating loss. Just because our society does not legitimize loss suffered from infertility and miscarriage does not mean it should go unacknowledged or that your pain is any less than if you had lost someone you loved.

Think about creating a ceremony that would help you say goodbye to the babies you lost, the cycles that failed, the opportunities you missed, and so forth. One couple collected rocks from a place that was special to them. They then buried them in their backyard, each one symbolizing an IVF cycle that failed. Another couple met with close friends and family over dinner and told them about their years of turmoil, their miscarriages, and their numerous failed attempts. Still another woman planted rose bushes along her driveway, one for each year she spent in treatment. Although these ceremonies were sad, they were also liberating, enabling couples to move on with their lives, either to create families in new ways or to feel resolved in their commitments to live child-free.

2. Shouldn't We Try Medical Treatment Just One More Time?

My husband and I want children very badly, but with my endometriosis and his low sperm count it seems as if it's going to take a miracle for me to get pregnant. So far we have tried every treatment the doctors have offered us, but nothing has worked. We're about to try our sixth IVF cycle, but to be honest we're not very hopeful anymore. I guess the thing that keeps us going back is that every time we try a cycle, the doctor seems to know more about what is happening and we seem to get closer to success. That makes us afraid to stop. What if we didn't do this cycle and this ends up to be the one that worked? I'm sure our doctor would tell us to stop if he thought there was no hope.

Like most people who experience infertility, you have put your reproductive life in the hands of your doctor. Handing over that much control to a health professional can eat away at patients' feelings of self-worth and helplessness. We know it is extremely hard for infertility patients to get off the medical roller-coaster, especially if their doctors are encouraging them by telling them the next treatment could be "the one." However, according to the literature we reviewed, most reproductive endocrinologists feel that success rates actually decrease after three or four IVF cycles. If the first attempt (which many physicians view as diagnostic) is not successful, then the second to fourth cycles involve perfecting drug dosage and techniques to optimize the chances of pregnancy. After that, the chance for pregnancy decreases.

You may begin to regain control of your treatment plan by questioning your doctor on exactly what he means when he says that each attempt is getting you closer to success. It would also be helpful to question him on his success rates and how many IVF attempts it normally takes for his patients to achieve full-term pregnancies.

In addition to feeling powerless, you say you are "afraid" to end medical treatment. And that, too, is an absolutely normal feeling. According to Susan Jeffers, Ph.D., author of *Feel the Fear and Do It Anyway*,[5] we can never escape the feeling of fear. No matter how hard we try to avoid feeling afraid, everyone feels afraid in moving forward with his or her life. What is important is how you view the fear. It sounds as if you are afraid of moving away from medical treatment because of the looming questions: Will this cycle be the one to get me pregnant? If I stop now, what if I miss my last chance at finally becoming pregnant?

You cannot answer these questions at this point. However, there is one question you do have to confront: *What if this cycle fails?* Answering this requires considering several other questions: Where will this cycle leave you financially? Given your history, you can probably evaluate whether or not you are prepared to endure the ups and downs again—do you have enough emotional and physical stamina to make it through? Have you explored other ways to create the family you long for?

Other people who have pursued medical treatment and eventually made the decision to end it have also experienced fear, but they have used the fear to motivate them to take action. They have turned around their negative feelings of being afraid into positive energy. Jeffers calls this "moving from pain to power."[6]

For a moment, try imagining that you really *do* have the power to create change. Imagine that you can redirect the same energy pushing you into the infertility clinic each month through another door that will give you more options.

If your fear is too giant a boulder to push aside, or if you cannot find the energy to motivate yourself toward change, we suggest you seek the help of an infertility or grief therapist. After a few sessions you may be able to look your fear in the eye and move on.

3. I'm Ready to Move On but My Wife Isn't

We have been trying to get my wife pregnant for the last four years. By "we" I mean me and an array of specialists. But with no luck. I am willing to walk away from the whole thing. So we don't have children. We have each other—isn't that enough? My wife walks out of the room whenever I try to have this conversation. You would think after four years my wife would begin to see a pattern here. Every month she can't wait for a new cycle to start. What are we going to do if she never wants to quit? Are we going to be the only sixty year olds at the IVF clinic?[7]

In the introduction to this chapter, we mentioned that there are two sides to the decision to end treatment; an emotional one and a logical one. Your wife may be making her decision to continue treatment based on her emotions, while you may be making your decision to end treatment based on logic. It is going to take time before some middle ground can be reached. Your wife will not be able to really hear you, until she feels ready to let go of having a biological child, and more importantly, to give up a part of her identity as a reproducing female. (See Chapter 1.) Likewise, you will have trouble understanding her until you can understand the feelings of loss you both might experience if you stop medical treatment.

You will need to *explore* each other's feelings about the situation so that you can reach some commonality. This involves communication. In *Sweet Grapes: How to Stop Being Infertile and Start Living Again* (Perspectives Press, 1989), authors Jean and Mike Carter advocate using *crisis communication* during crises. Couples have to find new and different ways to communicate while making the life-altering decisions you are about to make. Instead of talking to one another to convince or state positions, crisis communication involves *using words to explore your own feelings, testing new ideas and concepts, delving into what your partner is feeling, and sharing and working together to plan the future.* Guidelines for this form of communication include:

1. Be honest and forgiving. Since you are in the midst of making a major life decision, you will want to be as honest with your wife as you are with yourself. Don't worry about making a "good point"; instead concentrate on seeing whether each other's ideas might work for both of you. It is important to make allowances and not make your wife account for her feelings. Be forgiving of things she might have said to you during this stressful time as well as any inconsistencies in her argument.

2. It is okay for you and your wife to feel ambivalent because you are in a crisis. What you say or feel might not seem logical all the time. However, if you are there to listen and not immediately react negatively to each other, you will both be much freer to explore other options such as adoption, child-free living, donor options, and so forth.

3. Do not rest on assumptions—you may not know everything there is to know about each other's feelings. It is okay for husbands and wives to feel differently about their infertility; in fact, most do. The most crucial component of communication is understanding why your partner feels the way she does and accepting the fact that you do not agree. Simply validating each other will help to lessen the gap between the two of you.

4. Communicate in such a way that you both win and neither loses. Listen to each other and see if you can put yourselves in each other's position. Look for compatible feelings, such as: Are you both sick and tired of getting nowhere? or Do you both want to move on and don't know where to begin?

5. Allow for lots of time to explore each other's feelings. Your decision has to feel good to both of you, and that will take *many* thoughtful discussions.

4. I Want to Move on to Adoption but My Husband Doesn't

I'm about to undergo my fifth IVF cycle. We have also decided to apply to the donor embryo program at the clinic and place ads for adoption. We are not sure what is going to work for us, but we're so sick of waiting. I'm really ready to move on. I feel like I've let go of the idea of having a child that is genetically related to us. I know I want to become a parent no matter what. My husband's family thinks we're crazy and wants us to take one road at a time. They have been pressuring my husband so much that he's having second thoughts about placing the adoption ads. Last week he told me that he thinks we should wait until after we are done with the medical treatment. Since then we have been fighting about everything. I'm really not sure what to do anymore—we can't seem to agree and now both of us are miserable.

Although your husband's parents are voicing their concerns about your desire to pursue several options at once, it might be possible that your husband is not ready to move ahead as quickly as you are. Ending medical treatment and pursuing alternative ways to create families can be just as hard for a man as it is for a woman. Some men very much desire to experience a pregnancy with their wives and see what their offspring would be like. However, men typically do not voice these feelings believing they have to be strong for their spouses during the emotional ups and downs of the infertility experience. They can go for years without understanding their feelings about infertility until the point at which their wives want to end treatment. Then they are hit with the reality that they may never have a biological child. Because they have not had the time needed to grieve and let go of their dream, they are not ready to move on.

It is possible that your husband needs this grieving time now. Encourage him to talk. Let him know that you will not negate his feelings, even if you do not agree with him. He might need to hear *how* you came to decide to become a parent "no matter what." Also talk with other couples who have experienced a similar situation. Adoptive fathers are usually thrilled to talk about their feelings and will help both of you understand you are not alone. Be patient with your husband. He needs time and space to sort out his feelings.

5. Is It Possible to End Too Soon?

I have been a vegetarian since I was sixteen years old. Currently I exercise, meditate, and pride myself on staying physically fit and emotionally healthy. However, I have been unable to get pregnant for the past two years. The only thing doctors have diagnosed is mild endometriosis. My doctor believes I would have a good chance of getting pregnant if I went on Lupron for a few months, but after hearing about the side effects I don't think I want to. As one who rarely takes even aspirin,

I can't imagine taking such a risky drug. My husband and I are considering adoption instead, but friends, relatives, even members of my support group are trying to convince me that I'm quitting too soon. Now I'm not sure.

The decision about how long to stay behind the medical door is totally up to you and your husband, not your physician, friends, or family. Since most people experiencing infertility stay in treatment for years, the resistance you are getting may come from the fact that you have gone against the grain.

Physicians, especially those specializing in infertility, feel the use of drugs like Lupron or other similar medications are not potentially harmful. Apparently your physician views this drug as an effective way to cure your endometriosis. And even though there could be some side effects, your doctor believes the gain would outweigh the possible liabilities. However, he or she would not be the one experiencing these side effects. Only you and your husband can make this decision.

By using the word "quitting," your friends, family, and support group have placed a value judgment on your decision to end treatment. Many people expect an infertile couple to exhaust all medical options before adopting a child. They see adoption as the last choice rather than a viable alternative to having a biological child.

It is wonderful that you view adoption as a positive solution to your situation. But before pursuing this alternative plan, make sure you have grieved the loss of the reproductive experience. As Merle Bombardieri says,

> . . . allowing yourself to feel what you feel, to share it with your spouse, to comfort each other, and to share this sadness with others, is actually a way of gaining control. Letting it out allows it to come to an end, while pushing it down may sentence you to years of chronic depression. Once you've completed the grief process, you'll still have twinges of sadness about infertility, but you'll be ready to get on with your life.[8]

If, after future exploration of adoption, you decide to pursue medical treatment, you might want to approach your physician and see if you can come up with a mutually acceptable treatment plan. Some IVF clinics are willing to do a "natural" (drug-free) cycle. And some physicians advocate using acupuncture, herbs, and other forms of Eastern medicine to heal infertility. There are also treatment plans that include various forms of stress reduction to aid in the process of achieving a pregnancy. Taking your medical care into your own hands will lessen your anxiety and give you the sense of control you might be looking for at this time.

6. Are We Too Old to Start Medical Treatment?

Two years ago my wife had a miscarriage, and since then she hasn't been able to get pregnant. Our doctor is telling us to consider doing an IVF cycle. But because of our age—we are both forty-one—we're confused. Should we try medical treatment, or look into adoption? We definitely want to have a family.

You and your wife are ahead of the game by being certain that, no matter what, you want to be parents.

As we have advised other couples trying to make the decision about whether to end medical treatment or adopt, you first need to review the facts about your options. Since age does play a factor in the success rates of assisted reproductive technologies, you will have to ask your physician how she or he is going to optimize your IVF cycle. One physician we spoke with said that an IVF cycle in conjunction with ovulation induction and GIFT (gamete intrafallopian transfer) might increase the chances for success in women your age. However, if you are like some women over forty who do not respond well to ovulation induction treatment, there are other avenues to pursue. The use of a donor egg or embryo is another viable alternative, since it is the age of the egg that influences the outcome of the cycle. According to Carla Harkness in *The Infertility Book,* "with hormonal support, many women in good health can successfully carry a pregnancy through their forties and . . . even in their fifties. Using eggs donated from a younger woman increases the live, full-term birth rate for a woman over forty from less than 15 percent to more than 30 percent."[9]

If you decide to stick with an adoption plan, you will want to do some research before making any commitments to attorneys or agencies. There are many books available on the subject. Talk to other adoptive parents to understand the emotional and practical issues involved in adoption. Adoptive parents are usually thrilled to speak about the way their child(ren) came into their family and might be able to give you some pointers on how to make the process a little easier. Appendix II offers a list of support groups for couples interested in exploring adoption.

7. We Are Spinning Our Wheels

My husband and I have been undergoing infertility treatments for the past five years. Our diagnosis is male infertility. We have gone through four IVF cycles using micromanipulation and have had no success. We both want to end this part of our medical treatment but can't decide between adoption or donor sperm. How can we stop spinning our wheels and get on with our lives?

Your goal now is to narrow your field of options. Read as many books as possible about donor sperm and adoption. Find ones that not only give factual information but personal accounts as well. Check in with yourself as you read to see if you are experiencing any reactions, either positive or negative. Have your husband read the same books so when you are ready to talk, you can compare responses.

Another helpful way to gather information is to talk with other couples who have opted for either donor sperm or adoption. Your local RESOLVE chapter or adoptive parent support group will be able to provide you with names of people who feel comfortable talking about their choice. Ask each couple why they chose donor or adoption. How do they feel about their choice now? How are their friends and family responding to their choice? Once again, as you listen, notice your own positive or negative reactions.

After all these tasks are complete, the single most important thing to do is to allow yourself to visualize what life will be like as a parent. Can you see yourself with a child who comes to you either through adoption or donor sperm? Think about how it would be for you to not experience pregnancy, childbirth, nursing, and so on. How would it be for you to have a baby that is not genetically related to your husband, or one that does not have biological ties to either one of you?

Many people have told us that their visualizations gave them good feedback. They were able to understand which images were holding them back and which ones were pushing them to move forward. One woman who decided on adoption said that, before making her decision, she looked at other people's children at the mall, and tried to imagine loving them. But when she really looked at them, she realized her heart was open to loving any child. Then she knew her choice was right. You might want to try this as well as other visualizations (see Appendix I).

8. Medical Treatments Are Getting Too Expensive for Us

We have been going through infertility treatments for years, but inseminations and even Pergonal shots were covered by our insurance. Our insurance doesn't, however, cover IVF, which now seems to be the next step in our treatment and our last chance at having a biological child. Our doctor said we should plan on three cycles, but we just don't have the money.

We are sorry you have to make decisions regarding your health and your reproductive life based on money. Unless mandated by state legislatures, most insurance companies will not cover the high cost of assisted reproductive technologies. Unfortunately many legislatures do not understand the seriousness of infertility and have instead labeled it a "cosmetic" problem. This lack of acknowledgment by our government and the health care system in general is a blow to people already suffering from the devastating impact of infertility.

As more and more people are having trouble financing their infertility treatment, many couples consider the following to obtain the funds they need:

1. Borrow money from either a bank or family member.
2. Refinance your home.
3. Ask your doctor whether you can work out a budget plan with the office manager or participate in a research project.
4. Inquire about purchasing a rider to your insurance policy; check with your employer to see whether this is possible.
5. Consider changing to a job with a better health plan, assuming there are no restrictions on preexisting conditions.

We hate to see patients get themselves into debt or leave a job they like because of infertility. For approximately every twenty patients who get pregnant and give birth, there are another eighty who try it and do not. These are not great statistics, especially if you are borrowing money against them.

Of course, this is a logical answer for a very emotional problem. It is hard to have the decision made for you to end medical treatment. We hope you will consider looking at other ways to create your family, by adoption or deciding on child-free living.

9. We're Thinking about Adoption—Where Should We Start?

We are seriously considering ending medical treatment and moving on to adoption, but we don't have a clue as to where to start. Can you help us?

You will be confronted with many decisions during your exploration of adoption. Some, such as determining your financial limits, will be relatively straightforward, while others, like how much contact you will want to have with a birth mother, will require searching your soul. As you begin your research into adoption it will be helpful for both of you to keep in mind the following questions:

1. Do we want to adopt a newborn, toddler, or an older child?
2. Are we open to adopting a child who is not of our ethnic or racial backgrounds?
3. How many children are we willing to adopt at one time?
4. How much money can we reasonably allocate toward adoption?
5. Are we open to meeting a birth mother and possibly establishing a long-term relationship with her?
6. How long are we willing to wait for an adoption to occur?
7. Are we willing to reside in another country for an extended period of time in order to meet that country's requirements for finalizing the adoption?

In addition to looking at these issues, we suggest you also talk, read, attend lectures, go to support groups—do anything and everything that will give you access to the information you need to proceed. A good place to start is Appendix II. The adoptive parents organizations listed there can provide professional as well as personal insights into the emotional ups and downs surrounding the arrival of an adopted baby, and can recommend reputable adoption agencies and lawyers.

Aaron Britvan, an attorney who specializes in adoption law, says that couples need to find a qualified adoption attorney because

> although blissful in concept and simple in theory, adoption law is technical, inconsistent from state to state, and rife with procedural variations that cannot be ignored. A simple mistake could affect lives for many years and prove emotionally and financially costly.
>
> To the adopting couple, it may seem straightforward—locate an adoptable child through independent sources or an agency, and find a lawyer to handle the legal work. However, it's just not that easy. Couples in New York may want to adopt a California child, a California resident may seek a baby in Pennsylvania, a Pennsylvania couple may want an Arkansas adoption, or a couple from Washington, D.C. may be in search of a Korean child.[10]

No matter what route you pursue, be sure to obtain a qualified agency or lawyer who specializes in the type of adoption you are pursuing and who has a good reputation among other adoptive parents.

The following books will offer introductions to adoption:

• Bartholet, Elizabeth. *Family Bonds: Adoption and the Politics of Parenting.* Houghton-Mifflin Company, Boston, 1993.

- Johnston, Patricia. *Taking Charge of Infertility.* Pespectives Press, Indianapolis, Ind., 1994.
- Johnston, Patricia. *Adopting after Infertility.* Perspectives Press, Indianapolis, Ind., 1994.
- Melina, Lois. *Making Sense of Adoption: A Parents' Guide.* Harper & Row, Publishers, New York, 1989.

Good luck on your journey!

III

—

RESOLUTION

10

Child–Free Living
A Family of Two

I shall be telling this with a sigh
Somewhere ages and ages hence:
Two roads diverged in a wood, and I—
took the one less traveled by.
And that has made all the difference
—Robert Frost, from
"The Road Not Taken," 1916[1]

Couples living in today's world have more lifestyle options than ever before. This renaissance has made living without children a viable option for many couples whose interests are incompatible with raising children. Choosing a career over motherhood is no longer the unthinkable phenomenon it once was. Many child-free couples enjoy satisfying marriages, fulfilling careers, and active social lives. Yet infertile couples have difficulty accepting and sometimes even entertaining the thought of living child-free.

Studies show that part of the reason for this lies in the fact that although society has changed, the majority of couples today still conform to the traditional roles of provider and nurturer, even when the woman has a career of her own. This is not surprising since their feelings about parenthood are based on expectations laid down in early childhood. Most couples now experiencing infertility were raised during the 1960s and 1970s, a time when the male and female roles in households were clearly defined; it would have been very difficult to grow up during that period of time and *not* be influenced by these roles.

Therefore, couples experiencing infertility who avoid dealing with the subject of child-free living altogether may do so for a number of reasons. Some people believe that talking about living child-free will in some way jinx them or send a signal to God that they don't actually want children as much as perhaps another couple. Others believe such discussions will be too painful, and will bring up their worst fears of being forced into childlessness.

In order to even consider child-free living as a viable choice, infertile couples need to be open to looking back and reexamining why they wanted children in the first place. In doing so, some couples are surprised to discover that even after years of pursuing fertility, they now feel differently about becoming parents. If they have exhausted their emotional, physical, and financial resources, they may begin to see child-free living as a realistic and positive alternative to the life they once envisioned. When couples open their hearts to the idea that they can *choose* to be child-free, they are able to find new opportunities for growth and happiness, and can begin to live their lives again as a family of two.

Creating a new identity without children is the focus of this chapter. In it we discuss and answer questions regarding the task of becoming a *revised self.* This task is difficult for both partners who originally wanted to be parents, but it is especially difficult for women who have been taught that they were supposed to grow up and have babies.

When two people marry, the husband may work on his career and see himself as responsible for his wife's well-being. He may also anticipate and prepare for the fact that he will one day add to these responsibilities by becoming a parent. When a child does not arrive, the husband is able to maintain his work and continue to provide for himself and his wife. On a very practical level, child-free living means the husband remains responsible for two people instead of three or more. For some men this is somewhat of a relief. This is not to say, however, that men do not experience a great deal of loss when they cannot have children. The point is that even when a man does not have a child, his male identity remains intact. For some men the external pressures from wife, friends, or family to become a parent can be more difficult than their own feelings.

For women the task of coming to terms with and accepting their new identity as women without children goes against the grain of everything they have learned. Traditionally the only role models childless women had were the lonely old maids who lived down the street or the reclusive couples who wouldn't let children play in their yard because they didn't want their grass trampled on.

The times are changing, however. An increasing number of women are choosing to live their lives without becoming mothers. In 1994, according to the U.S. Census Bureau, women forty to forty-four years old, who represent the years of the baby boom generation, completed their childbearing years with childlessness levels of 18 percent, which was up from 10 percent in 1976. Women who were thirty to thirty-four and thirty-five to thirty-nine years old in 1994 and were near completing their childbearing years had levels of childlessness of 26 and 20 percent, respectively, each being about 6–8 percent higher than the levels recorded by women the same age in 1980.[2]

What all these numbers mean is that we, as a society, will collectively need to modify our view of women who are not mothers. In her best selling book *Women Who Run with the Wolves,* Clarissa Pinkola Estés, Ph.D., asks us to expand our definition of motherhood:

You are born to one mother, but if you are lucky, you will have more than one. And among them all you will find most of what you need. Your relationships with *todas las madres,* the many mothers, will most likely be ongoing ones, for the need for guidance and advisement is never outgrown, nor, from the point of view of women's deep creative life, should it ever be.[3]

This idea of needing more than one mother is important for all women to recognize, but it is especially significant for women who choose child-free living and still feel the need to nurture. Many women tell us of other women besides their own mothers who have had a positive influence in their lives. For some it was a grandmother, an aunt, a neighbor, a teacher or therapist, or even a mentor. *The capacity for a woman to inspire another's life is neither improved nor hampered by her ability to produce children.*

All children can benefit from having the guidance and support of many nurturing adults, both male and female. In African tradition there is a belief that it takes two people to bring a child into the world and a whole village to raise him or her. As one couple said, "Deciding to live child-free was difficult for us. But once we made the decision, we could turn our attention to our nieces and nephews. Now that our hearts are open to them, we have truly become their second parents. We are even thinking of volunteering at our church and running a support group for children whose parents are divorced. We want to be available to the children who need us."

As you will see when you read through this chapter that although it takes time and effort, couples deciding to live child-free can and will find their own special way of leaving their mark on the world.

1. Child-Free or Childless—Is There a Difference?

I always thought people who couldn't have children were childless. Now I hear people say they are living "child-free." What's the difference?

The difference between these two terms is enormous. Let's examine the two suffixes to the word "child": "Less" is defined as "with the deduction of; minus, or smaller." On the other hand, "free" is defined as "to set at liberty; make free, to relieve of a burden, obligation or a complaint."[4] What a difference a word makes!

Until recently our society has used the word "childless" to describe individuals and couples who for one reason or another lived without children. This word still conjures up images images of lonely old maids and reclusive couples. Women who were unable to become pregnant or carry a baby to term were described as "barren." Men without children were thought to be less of a man. Sadly, many people lived their lives with this negative identity.

"Child-free" is a relatively new term, coined by individuals who feel their choice of living without children is not as sad as stereotypes previously led people to believe. Instead, they see child-free living as a conscious and positive choice. They view their lives as pleasurable, gratifying, and productive. Jean and Mike Carter emphasize this point in their book *Sweet Grapes: How to Stop Being Infertile and Start Living Again:* "Childfree means turning involuntary childlessness into voluntary childlessness. And we would rather live our lives in the achievement of a major life goal than in the constant reminder of the frustration of one."[5]

2. Will Our Family Ever Understand?

My husband is an only child, and our decision to live child-free has created a lot of problems with his family. His mother is constantly making comments about how selfish we are for not giving her grandchildren, and his father keeps talking about how we have put an end to the family name. How can we get them to understand and accept our decision?

Handling the intense emotions of our parents is difficult at any age, but it can be especially difficult when you have just gone through years of a crisis and would like to feel acceptance from those closest to you. It is important to understand that your in-laws are probably dealing with their own sense of loss and need time to come to terms with the situation.

Like most other parents of adults, your husband's parents feel they are entitled to have grandchildren and hold their children responsible for fulfilling the dream. This is a heavy load for a person and unfortunately also an unspoken "understanding" in many families. Also, many times parents feel guilty when their children decide not to have children. They wonder what could have been so bad about their own parenting that their children would not want to become parents.

Make your in-laws aware of the pain and anguish you suffered when you were pursuing conception, and how and why you came to the decision to live child-free. You might also want to share any books or articles that you found particularly helpful in making your decision. Eventually you might even suggest that they express their grandparenting energies in other ways such as volunteering for charitable organizations like a foster grandparent program, or at a day-care center or hospital.

While not a complete substitute, it may be just what they need to satisfy their need to nurture.

By sharing this very personal and intimate experience with your husband's parents you pave the way to better understanding. This does not guarantee acceptance, but it can lead to more honest communication. Through patience and mutual respect you may be able to shape an entirely new relationship with them.

3. My Infertile Friends Aren't Supporting My Decision

When I was in the middle of my infertility treatment, I joined a support group. For the first time I felt like someone understood exactly how I was feeling. When the group ended two years ago we all remained friends and helped each other through treatments, pregnancies, and adoptions. At a recent meeting I announced that my husband and I have decided to stop trying to have a baby. As I explained to the group how we had come to this decision and our plans for the future, they all became unusually quiet. No one has said anything to me about our decision since that night. I don't understand their silence. I am starting to feel very alone again.

When you announced to your group that you and your husband have decided to live child-free, you undoubtedly expected them to be supportive and understanding. Their response did not meet your expectation, and you were understandably disappointed. Why is the subject of child-free living so taboo to your group?

When child-free living is discussed in support groups, some members become so uncomfortable, they try in every way possible to steer the conversation away from the subject. Since living without children is the outcome most feared by infertility patients, their response is not surprising. Those in your group who already have children might interpret your decision as either a threat or a devaluation of their choice to parent. Some may fear the loss of your friendship, believing their parenting stories will bother you. Others might feel jealous of the lifestyle you have chosen but are unable to admit it to themselves. Still, others will feel that even exploring child-free living as an option will jinx their ability to get pregnant.

It is no wonder that you are feeling isolated and abandoned again. It might be worth sharing your feelings of hurt, if these friendships are important to you. You may want to discuss the ways in which you have been able to integrate infertility into your identity, how you now feel open to experiencing life without the expected or assumed role of being a mother, how your horizons have expanded to include other visions of yourself and your husband. You are not alone in your chosen lifestyle. It has been estimated that 15 to 20 percent of the baby-boom generation born in the 1950s and early 1960s will remain child-free.[6] Bear in mind that the group's reactions to your situation might be similar to the reactions of other friends and family you choose to tell, so working this out with your support group will be good practice for other discussions.

Look for other available sources of support. Some infertility-related organizations provide education and support for people choosing child-free living. Many publish newsletters, plan social and educational events, and encourage their members to view life without children as a viable, acceptable way to create a family. If you found the infertility support group to be helpful before your decision, then you will probably also feel supported by a group for couples living child-free. One such organization is listed in Appendix II. If there are no groups in your area, Linda Anton in *Never to Be a Mother* suggests ways to begin a self-help group.[7]

4. Will We Have Regrets?

After fifteen years of marriage and ten years of infertility, my wife and I have decided to live without children. It took us a long time to come to this decision, but we finally realized we were leading very fulfilling lives. The problem is that everyone around us seems to think we will regret our decision when we are older. They say by the time we realize our mistake, we will be too old to do anything about it. Do you think we will regret our decision?

You might recall the book *The Road Less Traveled* by M. Scott Peck, which has been on the *New York Times* best-seller list for many years. One reason for its popularity stems from a desire many people have to further explore the roads and paths they chose to follow as well as those they were too afraid to take. In our society, many people live their lives assuming that those who take the road less traveled are doomed to fail or at least have regrets. This could explain why your friends and family feel so skeptical of your decision and why you are wondering whether you will look back with regret.

Perhaps your family and friends are more invested in your becoming parents than you realize. Some of them might have been looking forward to becoming aunts, uncles, or grandparents to your children and sharing parenting experiences with you. They may also be very confused about how you could come to this decision after so many years of wanting a child. Just as you needed time to let go of your dreams, so, too, do your family and friends.

To test your decision, try imagining your child-free life by using the visualization technique described in Appendix I. Imagine your life ten years from now. Where do you live? Are you happy? What do you do with your free time alone and together? Imagine yourself and your wife as senior citizens sitting quietly in a place that is peaceful and serene. Can you turn to each other and say, "Our life has been good. We've made some difficult choices and compromises, but we've done all or most of what we wanted"? Can you imagine feeling fulfilled?

As humans we are always struggling to figure out whether the decisions we have made were the right ones. We sometimes find ourselves fantasizing about the other possibilities, wondering if the grass would have been greener. For most of us, these feelings are short-lived. We leave our fantasies behind and return to our day-to-day lives. Although the pain of the past might creep in from time to time, it does not stop us from believing that the choices we have made are for the best.

Couples who have chosen child-free living after infertility report that they feel secure and comfortable with the decision, and that with time their friends and families have developed new attitudes.

5. I Just Can't Seem to Decide

For the past two years, my husband and I have seriously considered living child-free, but whenever I think about it, I'm just not sure. I find myself back in treatment, get frustrated again, and then begin to look into adoption. It's becoming a vicious cycle. I am an independent person, so sometimes the idea of living child-free is very appealing, but other times I think I would like a child to nurture.

The couples in your situation have been termed "drifters."[8] These are people who never decide to end medical treatment, never decide to adopt, and never decide to live child-free. They float along in an ambiguous state, allowing their infertility to control them. Almost all infertile couples experience drifting at some point during their infertility treatment; rather, it is those who never leave the vicious circle who get into trouble.

You sound as if you are ready to put an end to chronic drifting since you see yourself as an independent person. To see whether child-free living is right for you, try these steps:

1. Make a list of all the financial, social, emotional, and physical advantages of living without children. Ask your husband to do the same.
2. List some of the ways you fulfill your nurturing impulses in your everyday life. Many couples report finding meaning in other relationships with their

nieces and nephews, or with friends' children. Many volunteer for child-centered organizations. Others focus on their pets or gardens.

3. Consider committing yourself to a period of time in which you and your husband live as a child-free couple. That means stopping all medical treatment and inquiry into adoption. It may even mean using some form of birth control so that you will no longer have to wait to see if your period arrives or have to deal with incessantly wondering, "What if . . . ?"

4. During this time, socialize with other couples who have chosen this lifestyle. An organization listed in Appendix II can help you meet similar couples.

Now, let yourselves "off the hook": see if you can turn this feeling of being victimized by the infertility into a sense of surviving no matter what the odds. Imagine finally being free. After years of infertility, it might take you a while to feel comfortable around children again. However, most couples find that they are less anxious around children the more they become immersed in their child-free lifestyle.

6. Is There Life after Infertility?

After seven years of infertility I've had it with medical treatments. I don't want to adopt or use a surrogate to carry my baby. But I've never been much of a career woman. I was always sure I would get pregnant someday and planned on staying home with my children. Since that's obviously not going to happen, what am I going to do?

It is likely that as a very young girl you envisioned yourself in a more traditional adult role as a stay-at-home mom. However, your current situation does not fit into those early images of adulthood. The need to alter one's dreams because of unplanned events, such as infertility, can rock even the most secure person's sense of control. But it can also open doors to opportunities and challenges you might never have dreamed possible.

You have taken one of the most important steps toward a final resolution by eliminating the options you are uncomfortable with. Now your task is to rethink your identity by exploring the possibilities that exist for you in living without children. One way to begin your search for your new identity, or *revised self*, is through the self-empowerment process presented by Marcia Chellis in her book *Ordinary Women, Extraordinary Lives*. The five steps in this plan are accepting, networking, choosing, shifting, and mentoring.[9]

1. ACCEPTING

Accepting child-free living as a positive alternative is the hardest and the most time-consuming part of the self-empowerment process. Chellis explains the difference between acknowledgment and acceptance:

> Acknowledgment is admitting, being able to say something is true. Acceptance goes much deeper. Acceptance does not mean yielding or giving up or tolerating: acceptance means receiving on an emotional level what one admits to be truth on an intellectual level.

Accepting means that, although you realize you will not have children, you possess an inner belief that you will move on to create a different and equally satisfying life. It means accepting the fact that you have just as much value and worth as a woman now as you did when you envisioned yourself as a mother.

2. NETWORKING

Networking is a strategy that will help you move ahead. Personal networking means getting to know other couples who are living child-free. You may find these people through friends, family, or child-free organizations. Talking with other child-free women may help you to see the many positive aspects of your choice and to truly accept your decision.

Professional networking involves seeking out people doing the kind of jobs that may be of interest to you. Start by inquiring whether career counseling is available at your local library. A career counselor will give you interest inventory tests that will match your interests and talents with possible careers. The book *What Color Is Your Parachute?*★ is a helpful guide in discerning what career path might be best for you. Take a course in an area of interest. Turn an enjoyable hobby into a successful business. If being around children is still important to you, contemplate a career in day care, teaching, or counseling.

3. CHOOSING

Choosing involves using what you have learned through networking and putting it into action. You may choose to return to school or become an apprentice.

★ Richard Nelson Bolles, *What Color Is Your Parachute* (Ten Speed Press, Berkeley, Calif., 1996).

You may choose to use birth control to end the monthly question of whether you might be pregnant. Choosing to let go of these monthly ups and downs is a liberating experience: it confirms and solidifies the choice of child-free living and replaces the helpless feelings that come from infertility with a greater sense of control.

4. SHIFTING

Shifting takes place when thinking in choiceful ways becomes the norm. You no longer wait for things to happen. You automatically move ahead in positive ways. The key to shifting is to develop the belief that you have choices and are willing to explore what possibilities exist. It means shifting or reframing your earlier mind-set of motherhood and substituting it with the belief that you can be fulfilled in ways you never thought possible.

5. MENTORING

Mentoring gives you the opportunity to give back to others what has been given to you. Becoming an active member of an organization for couples living child-free is a great opportunity to show others what you have accomplished. In addition to helping others, mentoring reinforces the choices you have made.

7. Where Will We Fit In?

Living with infertility for over ten years has shown me that people without children don't fit in with their families or society. Even our "infertile friends" are all parents now. Now that my wife and I are coming to the conclusion that we want to live child-free, we are wondering if we will ever fit in anywhere or if we are destined to live as outcasts.

There is a world of difference between the way you are feeling and the way child-free couples view their social lives. Couples who feel as if they are outcasts see themselves as *childless* and in turn always feel less than their peers. They do not feel valued in their social circles and begin to isolate themselves from people who at one time in their lives they viewed as close, nurturing friends. While some childless couples are in fact confronted with prejudice and stereotyping from others, sometimes these feelings are self-imposed: their friends find themselves feeling uncomfortable around the couple not because they don't have children, but due to the couple's general sense of uneasiness.

There is no way to tell from your question how you and your wife are being viewed by your friends; therefore, the focus of our answer will deal with the way the two of you view yourselves. The fact that you use the words "destined to live as outcasts" tells us you see yourselves in a situation you have no control over. While it is true that the outcome of each medical procedure is out of your hands, you can regain control over your lives through the resolution of your infertility. By "resolution" we mean more than simply making a decision to do one thing or another; rather, it is about feeling good about the decision. To resolve your infertility you need to go through a grieving process, which will allow you to say goodbye to the children you will never have and help you give up your dream of becoming a parent. While it may feel like you have been mourning these losses throughout your infertility, it is clear you have not completed the final letting go that needs to happen in order for resolution to occur.

The way to begin this process is to talk about your feelings with each other. You may find yourself crying or screaming, but the ultimate goal is to release all those pent-up feelings from the past. Give yourself time to grieve; it will not happen overnight. If at any time you are not sure how to proceed or are uneasy dealing with these feelings, then we suggest working for a short time with a therapist experienced in infertility or loss.

Next, consider having a ceremony for your unborn and unadopted children, just as people do when they experience a more tangible loss. If you still have those old petri dishes from an IVF cycle or paperwork from your research into adoption, take the time to find an appropriate burial ground and say goodbye by burning or burying the remains of your infertility. Although this may sound extreme or dramatic, rituals similar to these have helped many couples feel less burdened and more open to the benefits of child-free living.

The final phase of letting go consists of hope and recovery, when you come to believe you are truly not destined to live as outcasts in society but as a family of two. In this stage you gain pleasure from seeing things differently and begin to feel just as whole as your friends with children.

As you move on in your life and incorporate the advantages of being a family without children, finding child-free people to socialize with will not be as difficult as you might imagine. It may be easier for you to develop friendships with couples who started having children early in their lives. By the time they are forty, their children are grown, and they resume a "child-free" lifestyle, with more time to spend with friends and fewer issues and responsibilities surrounding parenting. Organizations that cater solely to child-free couples like the Childfree Network (see Appendix II) are another good way to make friends who share your lifestyle.

Once you and your wife begin to embrace your new lifestyle, you can enjoy the company of nurturing friends who can be both sensitive to the years you spent in turmoil over infertility and supportive of your conscious decision to live as a child-free family.★

8. Can Our Marriage Survive without Children?

My husband and I have been living child-free for the past year, and everything seems to be going incredibly well. The emotional and financial stress of baby making is gone, and we are enjoying our marriage and our lives more than we ever have before. My only concern is whether it will last. Do marriages do well without children, or will my husband someday leave me for a woman who can give him a child?

For many years, people believed that a sure fix for an unstable marriage was having a baby. They thought that a child would guarantee a lifetime commitment. Not only was that theory incorrect, but we now know that the converse is actually true; research has shown that couples who have children report higher rates of marital satisfaction before they had children and again after their children leave home than while they are raising them.[10]

Your fear of your husband leaving you is common among infertile women. However, when both partners are equally satisfied with the resolution of their infertility, such fears are completely unfounded. Couples who have experienced infertility tend to "communicate better, share more opinions equally, and have fewer extramarital affairs than parents do."[11]

Infertility can help couples develop a strong, longlasting commitment to one another. Although infertility can wreak havoc on marriages, the majority of couples do stay married and use the lessons learned from infertility to guide themselves through future crises.

In order to feel secure in your commitment to each other, you and your husband need to view yourselves as a family and to establish your own rituals and traditions. Many couples believe in celebrating holidays in creative ways that

★ Linda Hunt Anton, *Never to Be a Mother* (HarperCollins Publishers, New York, 1992), pp. 89–92, discusses ways for women who didn't or couldn't have children to deal with their loss.

acknowledge and affirm their lifestyle. For example, many child-free couples have a yearly tradition of inviting friends and family to their homes, while others plan their yearly vacation around holiday time or focus their energies on a charity. But, most couples say they like to incorporate some of the customs from their families of origin so they can feel they are "passing the tradition on" to their partners.

Couples who opt not to have children in their families have the ability to take better care of each other. There is more freedom to travel and live spontaneously, and because of less financial strain, the couple has more options when choosing work schedules or careers.

9. What about Old Age?

If my wife and I do decide to live child-free, who will take care of us when we are too old to take care of ourselves?

This is a question we hear from almost every couple considering living without children, because like you they believe that children are guaranteed caretakers. However, studies have shown that having children does not provide the emotional or custodial security needed in a couple's senior years.

Susan Lang, who thoroughly researched this topic in *Women without Children,* found that the role of adult children in their parents' lives is not what we would expect. "Seniors with children do, in fact, have frequent contact with their adult children—about seventy five percent of older persons see one child at least weekly. Yet several studies suggest that there's little, if any, link between an elderly parent's contact with his/her grown children and their morale." Lang encourages the development of strong social support. In her interviews she found that "the number of friends a senior has is not the critical factor for emotional well-being. . . . What's most important is having *at least one* confidant."[12]

Since we live in an ever-changing society, where family members no longer feel obliged to stay close either physically or emotionally to each other, seniors will be forced to find new and innovative ways to take care of each other in their golden years. One solution is the formation of adult communities, which are becoming more and more common. Many gerontologists, who study aging and the elderly, believe that these supportive environments will allow senior citizens a longer period of independence.

The other key to success in old age is to plan ahead and provide for any unforseen crises. The Carters suggest in *Sweet Grapes: How to Stop Being Infertile and Start Living Again* that child-free couples take the money they would have spent on children and save it to avoid financial problems that could compromise their health or housing.[13] Thinking about where you would like to live after you retire is also a good idea. Keep in mind that your support network will probably be the most important source of your companionship.

10. My Husband Wants to Live Child-Free and I Don't

My husband and I got married when we were both in our thirties. Because of this time factor, we wanted to have children right away. After trying everything to get pregnant, including three unsuccessful IVF cycles, we decided to look into adoption. My husband was reluctant, but went along with it because of me. After six months of trying to adopt a baby, my husband laid down the law and said, *"no more!"* He is tired of having our whole life revolve around getting a baby. So now I have to choose between my husband and a baby. I know my decision will be to stay married, but what will I do if I keep wanting to have a baby?

When men are very reluctant to parent, the situation does not resolve itself when the baby arrives. Often what happens is that the husband does not contribute to the caretaking of the child and his wife ends up feeling alone and angry. Something that they both worked so hard for ends up backfiring.

However, we do not think your husband is merely reluctant to parent, nor do we think he has run out of patience in trying to have a child. His initial hesitancy to adopt and the fact that you went through years of infertility yet only tried adoption for six months indicate that the real issue is adoption. For his own reasons your husband is unable to accept an adopted child as his own.

Considering your husband's objections, we support your decision to live child-free. However, making this choice does not mean your work is over. We suggest making an appointment with a marriage counselor well versed in infertility issues, so you and your husband can talk about all your feelings in a supportive environment. This will also give you the opportunity to work through any anger or resentment you have toward your husband or the situation you have found yourself in. Open communication is absolutely critical to your marriage. If your husband is unwilling to see a therapist, then you can still benefit from going yourself.

Giving up your dream of children for the sake of your marriage will take a heroic effort, but it is possible. We recently spoke with a couple who had been in a situation very similar to yours. The husband felt that if he could not have a biological child, he would prefer to remain child-free. After reexamining his decision in counseling, he found that, although he wanted to please his wife, he could not change his feelings enough to be comfortable with adoption. His wife was very angry and wondered if she would ever be able to forgive him. At one point, she even thought about leaving him to become a single parent. Over time she realized that the anger she felt was not totally due to her husband's reluctance to adopt. The anger she had directed toward her husband slowly became refocused on deeper issues—the loss of her fertility and a baby.

Months later, when she was finally able to talk to her husband about her pain, he was also ready to express his sadness and guilt over the situation. It seems that he had never been really sure about his desire for a biological child and was almost sure that he could not give any child, especially one not genetically related to him, the kind of love and attention he felt was important. Moreover, she came to realize that her marriage was the greatest source of satisfaction in her life. Like you, she had waited to get married and felt her husband was truly the man she wanted to grow old with. Finally, their true feelings had emerged, so they were able to come to terms with each other and with living child-free.

As this situation highlights, a successful outcome is possible if you are willing to look at your loss and acknowledge it as a real and tangible feeling. *You will have to give yourself the time to actually be in pain* about what you have given up. In our society, we are encouraged to try to find band-aids to make our hurts get better quickly and easily. This will not work for you. The risk you take by not allowing yourself to get in touch with these "ugly" feelings is a lifetime of resentment toward your husband.

In *Never to Be a Mother,* Anton suggests that women in your situation have an *imagined* dialogue with the person they blame for their childless situation. You play both parts by writing down or saying what you believe to be true for both of you. Imagine the internal struggle of the other person as well as your own. The purpose of this exercise is to take blame out of the picture and replace it with forgiveness.[15] When you understand better the reasons why your partner has chosen not to parent, you may be able to live happily with your decision.

11

Waiting for Your Baby
Adoption and Pregnancy

Dear Baby,

I remember playing house when I was a little girl and stuffing a pillow under my shirt so I could look pregnant. I thought it was the coolest thing in the world to pretend to have a big belly and waddle around. I played and played with the baby dolls my mom brought me. I remember she used to tell me that the most important job in the world was to be a mom. When I married your dad, I dreamed of you every night. I imagined what you would look like. I even came up with names for you. I wanted you so badly, baby. I wanted the baby your daddy and I would make from our love, our commitment to each other, and our future. But it wasn't so easy. We went to doctor after doctor and nothing worked. I took drugs—your dad gave me shots every night. I went through three surgeries. I thought I would never be able to have a baby. And I was very, very sad.

But one day, I learned that I was pregnant. I was so happy. I called your grandparents and all your aunts and uncles. I thought I would love this experience, but I have to be honest with you, it hasn't been easy. Having you inside of me is so scary and so frightening that I call your dad at work every few hours wanting him to tell me that you and I will be all right. I feel so guilty about this. I wanted to enjoy this pregnancy, but now I can't wait till you are born, so I can finally be rid of this anxiety and just hold you and love you.—Mommy

Dear Baby,

After all the years of waiting for a baby, the call we got from your birth mother last week choosing us to be your parents made us happier than we've ever been in our whole lives. I couldn't believe our luck. Finally we found you, the baby that was supposed to come into our lives.

Waiting for you is the hardest thing we've ever done. I'm a wreck. I can't eat, I can't sleep, and I can't remember what I am doing half the time. People talk to me and I forget to answer them. I'm so scared that your birth mother will change her mind. I want so much to buy you everything you'll need. I want to paint your room and pick out just the right wallpaper and curtains, but I don't dare. I have tried to shop for you, but it's too hard, too scary. What if things don't go the way we desperately want them to? How could we go on? I want you to know how much we love you already, and how much we pray for your arrival. I just want to hold you, my baby, and love you forever.—Mommy

These are the voices of mothers in waiting. Although one is biologically pregnant and the other is adopting, they are *both* pregnant—with the anticipation of one of the most important events of their lives. Finally after all the failed attempts a baby is within reach. As excited as they are about the upcoming event, they are also filled with the fear and mistrust that once again something might go wrong.

If you are a parent in waiting, you know what we mean. Most of us who go through infertility are led to believe that once we get pregnant, or decide on adoption or third-party reproduction, we will be set free from the turmoil, fear, and the pain infertility has brought us. But waiting for your child will most likely not be easy. It is an experience like no other: stuck between the years of infertility and the creation of a new family.

Both of us remember so clearly those feelings of vulnerability, skepticism, and fear. What if we made a mistake? What if something goes wrong? We could lose the baby we longed for and the dream once again. The negative, pessimistic voice in our heads, which had grown louder and stronger over the years of struggling with infertility, told us not to get our hopes up, not to count on things working out. At some point in our past we each learned to trust that voice, believing it would protect us against further disappointment.

In this chapter we share stories of people who are still hearing that voice, still feeling afraid that something is bound to happen. Waiting for your child to be born demands taking a leap of faith. Part of that leap is letting go of the belief that thinking negatively will cushion any disappointments. Another part of that leap is trusting that you have done everything you could to ensure that the outcome will be successful: things such as finding a doctor who is supportive of you and familiar with infertility; finding a lawyer, agency, or third party who believes that walking the straight and narrow path is better than cutting corners to get a baby. And making that leap means trusting you can survive anything. Think about all you have been through already—all the failed treatments, the ups and downs, the losses. You have survived. You certainly will survive again, no matter what. Eventually most pregnancies after infertility work out, and if handled correctly most adoptions work out as well.

ADOPTION

1. Our Families Don't Want Us to Adopt a Baby from a Foreign Country

My wife and I had been going through infertility for five years when we decided we just didn't want to do it anymore. So we made plans to adopt a child from Mexico. We were very happy to have finally moved on, and felt a sense of accomplishment when we handed in all the paperwork. Unbeknown to us, however, our parents on both sides had been talking behind our backs, looking for a way to discourage us from "adopting a child who couldn't possibly look like us." They took Thanksgiving dinner to make their feelings known. They felt that "these" children, as they put it, came from "questionable backgrounds" and that heredity is much more important than we realize. There was shouting and a lot of things said that shouldn't have been. The worst of it is that now our child will have grandparents who obviously don't want them in the family. I'm not sure, short of disowning our families, how this will work out. Their attitudes will always be in the backs of our minds.

Despite what you have told your parents about your medical odds or any other aspects of your reality, they may still be holding on to the dream of a biological grandchild. Remember how hard it was for you to let go, to say goodbye to your dream of pregnancy and genetic offspring, in order to make room in your hearts for adoption? They too have to mourn the loss of a biological descendant. Help them by explaining the process you went through in order to let go of your original dreams and embrace new ones. If you do not feel comfortable doing this face to face, write a letter explaining your feelings. Enclose a RESOLVE pamphlet written specifically for family and friends of infertile couples. The Long Island, N.Y., chapter of RESOLVE has a video (available for purchase) geared toward educating and raising the consciousness of friends and family of the infertile.★

Your parents may be responding from ignorance. How many families do they know of who have adopted a baby from another country? Most likely, not many if any at all. Because of this, they may assume they would never be able to accept or love a baby of another race and culture.

Consider exposing them to families that yours will resemble. The agency you

---

★ Contact the national RESOLVE headquarters for both of these items; their address is in Appendix II.

are adopting from most likely has a list of adoptive parents you can call. Or you can invite your parents to attend a meeting of your local adoptive parents organization (listed in Appendix II). The more exposure you give them, the more their assumptions will be challenged.

One grandmother of an adopted Korean baby, who was originally opposed to her daughter's plans for an international adoption, said,

> I hardly knew anyone who adopted children, let alone a Korean child. I'd seen families like that in the grocery store, and I always wondered why they chose a child that looked nothing like them. So I was very leery at first. When my daughter told us about her intentions, I thought she was crazy for bringing more problems into her life. But when I saw how much she loved the baby and how much joy he brought to my daughter and son-in-law—really to all of us—I had no choice. I fell totally in love with my grandson. Now, if anyone dares to say anything negative about him, I am like the grandmother lion, the first to come to his defense.

Like this woman, most adoptive grandparents who were not supportive initially do change their minds. Many of the families who put up the biggest fights become the strongest advocates for out-of-race placements or international adoption.

2. Adoption Advertising Feels Awkward to Us

We want to adopt a child, and our lawyer told us to put ads in the paper to find a birth mother. The problem is, when our son or daughter is old enough to be told about where they "came from," we are afraid that telling them they came from an ad in a newspaper will give them the wrong impression. We feel strange placing our ads next to ads for used cars, so how are they supposed to feel good about it?

Most experienced adoption attorneys will tell you that the first step toward adopting independently is to make contact with as many people as possible. In your case, placing ads in newspapers, in states where independent adoption is legal, accomplishes just that and is actually quite ingenious. Women who are unsure about their pregnancies can look through their local paper in the privacy of their own homes and decide, without any pressure, who they want to call and interview as prospective adoptive parents. The relationship that develops from those phone calls can become the makings of the story you will tell your child about his or her adoption. Even though right now you don't have the exact words to go with this story, when the time is right you will find a way to express your feelings.

Here's what one adoptive parent told her thirteen-year-old daughter:

> The best way to reach women who were considering placing their babies with adoptive families was to place ads in as many newspapers as I could. We were very lucky, because after advertising for eight months your birth mother read our ad and decided to give us a call. I remember hearing her voice for the first time. I remember thinking this could be it, my prayers could finally be answered. We talked for a long time that day. I learned all about her and she about us. We will always feel very lucky and grateful that your birth mother read our cries for a child and knew deep inside her that it was best for you, for her, and for us to be your parents.

See whether this new way to look at advertising feels right to you. If not, consider agency or international adoption as possible avenues to pursue, since they will not require you to do any advertising.

By choosing the route most comfortable for you, you increase the chances that your child will be comfortable with it too.

3. My Wife and I Disagree about Whether to Adopt

About a month ago my wife and I decided we had had enough of medical treatment. We looked at all our options and decided to move on to adoption. Last week we met with an excellent lawyer, who is supposed to be the best in his field. He has been handling adoptions in our community for many years. When we went to him, we were very optimistic and sure about our decision, but now I am thinking we made a mistake. Unfortunately my wife doesn't agree. She doesn't seem to care about all the negatives he presented to us, like having to be fingerprinted and undergoing a home study to see if we would be good parents. He also said that if we did manage to find a birth mother, she would basically be calling all the shots. I have watched those news reports where they have taken children away from their adoptive parents. I don't know if I can go through with this, but my wife wants no part of my apprehensions. Whenever we talk about it, we fight. I don't know what to do.

An infertile couple usually experiences a great sense of relief when they decide to end medical treatment and move on to adoption. But when one partner waivers, it can feel as if the progress that has been made is lost. They become polarized as one tries to convince the other of the negatives and the other fights for the positives. (See Chapter 3 for help with communication.)

As you fight against adoption outwardly with your wife, you are probably feeling the same kind of struggle within yourself. One part wants to adopt a baby, and the other part feels apprehensive of the requirements and risks. Take a good look at the reasons for these requirements and at the actual risks involved.

Fingerprinting, home studies, and interviews can be imposing. But as time-consuming and ridiculous as they may seem, they are absolutely essential to keeping adoption legal. These requirements protect both the permanency of your child in your home and the rights of the birth parents. Although some couples try to circumvent the process, Aaron Britvan, an experienced New York state adoption attorney, says, "Too many individuals proceed in their quest for adoption with hardened feelings of desperation—seeking the 'quick fix.' Successful adoptions arise from taking the straight and focused road with no shortcuts. *Done legally, adoptions will, most times, work out.*"[1]

As with infertility, there are financial and emotional risks with adoption, and no guarantees. Cases like the ones involving Jessica DeBoer and Baby Richard are not the norm. The media focuses on the adoption-gone-awry stories, not the thousands of successful adoptions that take place each year.

Search your soul to see what is blocking you. Consider the words of Carlos Castaneda, who wrote in *The Teachings of Don Juan:*

> Look at every path closely and deliberately. Try it as many times as you think necessary. Then ask yourself and yourself alone one question. This question is one that only a very old man asks. My benefactor told me about it once when I was young and my blood was too vigorous for me to understand it. Now I do understand it. I will tell you what it is: Does this path have a heart? If it does, the path is good. If it doesn't it is of no use.[2]

Right now, you and your wife need some time out from the urgency to push ahead in order to really explore your feelings. Spend some time in the library reading books on adoption, or talk to other adoptive parents about their experiences.

4. What Do You Say to a Birth Mother?

The phone is in, the ads are placed, and my husband and I are anxiously awaiting our first call. *Help!* Is the phone really going to ring one day? If it does, what do we say, how do we act? Is there any way to prepare ourselves for these conversations?

Do you remember waiting for the phone to ring from a guy you had a wild crush on? What you probably didn't realize was that the boy at the other end of the phone was nervous too. The same is true for a birth mother. If she is serious about placing her baby, she will want you to accept her as much as you want her to like you.

When that phone finally does ring, you and the birth mother will probably both be in an extremely heightened state of anxiety. What do you say? The first rule is to go slowly. Let her set the pace. If she is reluctant to talk, you can start the conversation by asking her nonthreatening questions such as: where do you live? how old are you? and do you have any brothers and sisters? You can also ask whether she has any questions about you, or offer her some general information. Here is one woman's account of talking with potential birth mothers:

At first I was so nervous. Whenever the phone [rang,] my heart would pound, I felt like I couldn't breathe, and I could barely remember my name much less carry on an intelligent conversation. It took a few calls before I calmed down. Realizing that every phone call was not necessarily "the one" actually took some of the pressure off, although it never got easy. I also started using my "list," things about myself and my husband that I would want a birth mother to know, but were likely to forget in all the anxiety of trying to make a good impression. I wrote down that we had a big backyard with lots of trees, a close family, and that I would be staying home with the baby as a full-time mom. These were the kinds of things that I would want to know if I was choosing adoption for my baby— so I hoped the birth mother would like them too. We didn't offer a lot of details [just] pretty general things—but enough so that she got to know a little about us. People told us not to do [this], told us to wait for questions from her. They worried that we were running the risk of saying something a birth mother wouldn't like. But we felt it would be much better to know if we were compatible up front rather than months down the road. It just felt better to be honest."

Usually, as time goes on and the number of conversations increases, so does the amount of information exchanged. Some birth mothers prefer not to speak directly to adoptive parents. They may be feeling intimidated, guilty, or just plain shy, or they may prefer not to develop a personal relationship with the adoptive par-

ents. Respect her wishes. You can always ask a third party such as an adoption attorney, social worker, friend, or family member to act as an intermediary.

There are some very important questions you need answers to concerning the
birth mother's health, the birth father's health, their family backgrounds, and the
probable costs of the pregnancy including her medical and housing fees. These
questions can best be asked by your lawyer who will request necessary reports
from the providers of services.

Keep notes of your talks with the potential birth mother as well as a list of
questions that might come up in between conversations. Adoptive parents have told
us this helps them keep track of important information. Also talk to other adoptive parents about their phone conversations with birth mothers. Although every
situation is different, you might be able to get some good advice from their experiences.

5. How Much Is Too Much Contact with a Birth Mother?

The birth mother we are working with is in her eighth month of pregnancy.
For the last two months the only contact we had with her were weekly phone calls.
Suddenly she has decided she wants me and my wife present at the birth. This just
may be more than we can handle and certainly is more than we agreed to initially.
If we agree to be in the labor room, then what about after the baby is born—how
much contact will she want then? It's beginning to feel like our baby is being held
hostage and won't be released until we've met the demands of the birth mother.

I think we need to look for another situation; my wife, however, is adamant.
She says we've come too far to quit and need to stick with this till the end, even if
it's not what we had planned. Do you have some insights that could help my wife
see how risky this is getting?

Preadoptive situations always require the prospective parents, as well as the birth
parents, to take emotional risks. It comes with the territory. Both adoptive and birth
parents are torn between wanting to do what is best for the baby and what feels
right to them. Deciding whether to be in the delivery room with the birth mother
is one of those precarious decisions. Who would it be best for—you, the birth
mother, the baby? Before you decide whether the birth mother's requests are too
risky, consider the situation from her point of view and then maybe you will be
able to work with her again.

The decision-making process for a birth mother is usually so fraught with
confusion and intense emotion that she cannot possibly anticipate what her needs

will be at each stage of pregnancy. When you first spoke to the birth mother two months ago, labor and delivery were probably the last thing she wanted to think about. But now the date looms large, and she has no choice: she is forced to deal with it. As you can imagine, the circumstances surrounding the delivery of this baby are most likely not what she wanted for herself, especially if this is her first birth experience. She is probably scared and feeling very alone. If so, then she would want to have someone she knows and is comfortable with by her side. But she has chosen you. Why? Perhaps she does not have a mother or sister or close friend who can be there for her. Or perhaps she believes that the baby's parents would want to participate in the baby's birth and that you would want to support her. Try to consider these possibilities as her reasons for asking you to be in the delivery room.

Some adoptive parents who agreed to give the birth mother this kind of support have called it the most profound experience of their lives; watching their baby being born was an opportunity not to be missed. They would tell you that to hold your child seconds after its arrival will be a gift etched in your minds forever.

Other adoptive parents have told us a different story. They say they were uncomfortable sharing such an intimate experience with a birth mother. They would rather have stayed in the waiting room and had their first moments with their child in private, not with the birth mother, the physician, and the nurses watching. Even though their emotions were soaring high, and they held the baby in their arms, gave him or her the first kiss, their minds were begging them to not let go and trust that this was truly their child until the birth mother had signed on the dotted line.

In addition, some adoptive parents have told us that even meeting the birth mother posed a problem for them. After their babies came home, the parents could not stop seeing the birth mother's face in their minds. Most couples report, however, that the image of the birth mother fades as their children grow and take on their own personalities, styles, and looks.

Since the trend today is toward openness in adoption, there will no doubt come a time when such practices (such as meeting birth parents) will be studied as thoroughly as the implications of closed adoptions have been. Until that time prospective adoptive parents like you and your wife will have to rely on your instincts to tell you whether you wish to be present at the baby's birth. We hope you will be able to mutually agree on what to do. However, if you find yourselves in a stalemate—you not wanting to participate but your wife willing to—there are other options. Perhaps your wife can be with the birth mother while you wait "outside." There is no rule that says you must both be there.

Another alternative is to arrange for someone else to be with the birth mother in the delivery room. Your lawyer's office might be able to put you in touch with a counselor whose role would be to offer support to the birth mother and to negotiate future arrangements with her. It is important, however, to choose a counselor both knowledgeable about and supportive of adoption, and who will look out for the best interests of all the parties involved, especially those of the baby.

6. No Contact with the Birth Father—What Should We Do?

We have been working with a birth mother for four months, and she is due in three weeks. She is an answer to our prayers: a college student who comes from a good family and is not interested in parenting a child right now. We met with her a few times face to face and developed a nice relationship, warm and respectful. She has talked to our lawyer, who is also impressed with her.

But she has split up with her boyfriend who is the biological father of the baby, and wants nothing to do with him. Our lawyer is advising her to tell him of the pregnancy so he can sign the appropriate legal papers. But she refuses because she is afraid his parents would try to stop the adoption. We are afraid that if we take the baby, the birth father will come back and claim that his rights were not upheld. What should we do?

It is smart to question the rights of the birth father. Anyone pursuing an adoption should take all the necessary precautions to secure the permanency of their future family. This means that your lawyer, whom we assume is well versed in the field of adoption law, should ensure the rights of both you and the birth parents. You can determine whether your lawyer's advice seems comfortable to you by familiarizing yourself with your state's adoption law regarding its provision for birth fathers. The birth mother should also be encouraged to have her own legal representation. She might be more open to hearing about the seriousness of contacting the birth father from her own lawyer.

Amy Rackear, C.S.W., in an interview with a couple whose son's adoption was being challenged by his birth father, made the following recommendations: in addition to obtaining competent counsel,

1. Learn as much as you can about the birth father.
2. Make sure that a lawyer is present when the birth parents sign the surrender documents.

3. Research all jurisdiction issues, if any other state is involved.
4. Clarify who is responsible for financing the defense of a challenged adoption when an agency participates—you or the agency?
5. Consider purchasing an insurance policy that covers litigation costs.[3]

As stated throughout this chapter, creating a family by any means has its risks. Though we hear of families being split apart by the courts, the reality is that adoptions are rarely contested. "In the absence of empirical data, Susan Freivalds, the executive director of Adoptive Families of America, estimates that 30,000 adoptions of healthy babies under the age of two are processed annually. 'Our office,' says Ms. Freivalds, 'only hears a dozen or so per year that are going to court.' "[4]

7. What Should I Tell Relatives about Our Baby's Birth Parents?

When my mother called the other day and said she was planning a Fourth of July family reunion, I was ecstatic. After all these years, I meant what I said when I replied, "Yes, we would love to come." For the first time in so long, I visualized myself actually having fun. When I walked into the party, everyone would ooh and ah over how beautiful my baby was. I thought that I could finally feel comfortable with all my pregnant cousins and their children. We went to the party yesterday and of course everyone oohed and ahed and thought my daughter was cute. My husband and I walked around for a while with our chests puffed out, and it felt *soooo* good.

But, what I was totally unprepared for was my response when my cousins started asking me questions about her "real parents." They wanted to know if we knew who they were, how old they were, and why they had to give her up. They just couldn't understand how anyone, no matter the situation, could ever give up a child. One cousin even told me that now that we've adopted, "you'll get pregnant and have one of your own."

I stood there with my mouth hanging open, unable to say a word. Couldn't they see that I already had a baby, that I didn't want any other except the one I had? How could they have been so cruel? All I wanted to do was go home and call my friends who understood how lucky and blessed I felt to have the baby I had. How could I have been so naive to think that everyone would just accept our situation?

After all those years of waiting to enjoy your baby, it is a shame that the day you had envisioned was ruined by a few people. If you understand why they might have said the things they did, you may be better prepared to communicate with them in the future.

Most people do not know the adoption terminology. Usually they use words like "real parent," not to make you feel unreal or to negate your role in your child's life, but because they do not know the best words to use. From time to time you will have to educate those around you. Pat Johnston's work may be of help in this. As an author and publisher of numerous books about adoption, she has come up with a *positive adoption language* (PAL) list. Copies are available at no charge from Perspectives Press (see Appendix II). In addition, *ADOPTALK,* a publication of the New York State Adoptive Parents Committee, offers the following guidelines when speaking or writing about adoption:

- Never mention adoption unless it is truly relevant.
- "Real" and "natural" should not be used in reference to an adoptee's birth parents. Instead use "birth parent," "birth mother," "birth father," or "biological parent."
- "Own" should be used carefully. A child who is adopted by an individual is that individual's "own" child. It is inappropriate to differentiate between an adopted and biological child by labeling only the biological child as being his or her parents' "own child."
- Do not qualify a parent who adopts a child as an "adoptive parent." Simply state the relationship as "parent," "mother," or "father" (unless the biological parents are also mentioned, and confusion would result).
- Do not say, "The birth parent *gave up* the child for adoption." Instead say, "The birth parent decided not to parent the child."
- Like birth, adoption is a once-in-a-lifetime experience. Therefore, if the need ever arises to show how a child came into a family, say, "Mary was adopted," just as you would say, "Mary was born."[5]

Many people have trouble understanding how birth parents can choose not to parent the child they give birth to. Being able to make the best interests of the child paramount is not something many people would or could do. The next time someone questions the actions of the biological mother, it may help you to answer honestly with such statements as "She was very young and financially unable to care for a child at this time." If you are not up for a long explanation, you could say, "I don't really know, but I thank God everyday that she did."

Similarly, in most cases people do not say "You'll get pregnant now that you've adopted" to slight the value of the adopted child, but because it has happened to some adoptive parents they know or have heard about. However, it happens not because there has been an adoption, but because of the 5 percent spontaneous pregnancy rate among infertile couples who do not seek medical treatment. You may want to share these facts.

No matter what people say or ask you, the way you respond and how much information you share with them *is* always up to you. It is never necessary to answer every question. You will, as time goes on, become more experienced in your responses and be able to determine and sense at a moment's notice what feels appropriate to respond to and what does not. Be patient with yourself and with others. This is a brand new experience for all of you.

8. When Should We Tell Our Son about His Adoption?

My friends who have read everything there is to read about adoption tell me that I should be talking to my three-year-old son about his adoption. They think the earlier I say the words, the easier it will be for him to accept the fact that he was not born to us. They also tell me I should speak to him about his birth mother so he can be introduced to the fact that she exists. They say that the more we speak openly about her and the adoption, the more comfortable we will all be with the subject.

I really don't feel he is ready yet. He still has a hard time understanding simple concepts. I would feel guilty if I did not really think this through thoroughly and do what is best for him. What do you think?

Part of the difficulty parents and professionals have had in determining when exactly to tell a child about adoption stems from the fact that

> there are countervailing forces. One is that it should be early enough so that a child first hears it directly and lovingly from his or her parent(s) rather than from neighbors, relatives or siblings. On the other hand, there needs to be no rush developmentally. Recent research suggests that most children cannot grasp the meaning of adoption until [they are in] the age range of 5 to 7.[6]

And even though a majority of today's parents are telling their children about adoption early on, one of the largest and most comprehensive studies ever done on adoption found that "whether adoption disclosure is better at age 2 or 3 than at age 5, or 6, or even later probably depends on a wide range of factors. In terms of long-term mental health, it does not seem [to be] a factor."[7]

In the book *Communicating with the Adopted Child,* Miriam Komar, D.S.W., suggests there are

> three specific issues of intellectual comprehension that should be established before a child is ready for learning about adoption. They are:
>
> 1. the concept of the family unit to which the child belongs;
> 2. the recognition that families, and individuals exhibit differences; and
> 3. an understanding of human reproduction and birth.[8]

No gauge of when to tell a child about adoption is more important than a parent's own instinct. Parents who can put aside their own anxieties about "telling" and judge their child's readiness based on their knowledge of that child will make a better decision than if they rigidly follow the advice of any friend, book, study, or professional.

Even before your child is ready to be told about his adoption, it is a good idea for you and your husband to plan exactly what you want to say and how you want to say it. Then when the opportunity arises, you will be more comfortable with the discussion. Some parents find it helpful to write down the words first, to make sure they are age-appropriate for their child and truly express how they feel. Others believe in making a storybook about their child's adoption. If you choose to make a book you could include pictures of your son's homecoming and other special times you have shared. You may also want to add writings from your family and friends about what his arrival meant to all of you.

Remember, this is just an introduction to the concept. As your lives move on, your son will have deeper and more profound questions. He is still very young, so your current goal is to anchor him into your family by emphasizing how much you love him now and forever.

PREGNANCY

9. Pregnancy Isn't What I Expected

After trying to get pregnant for seven years, it finally happened. I guess I should be happy but I'm not. All day long I am terrified of losing this baby—which is why I don't want to get attached. There just isn't any guarantee that things will work out.

I haven't told many people, I would rather they not know just in case. My husband keeps telling me everything is going to be okay, but he doesn't know that. It seems so horrible that after all this time of trying to get pregnant, it has not turned out the way I envisioned it at all. It's nerve-wracking and upsetting and not much different than my experience with infertility. How am I going to get through this?

We have run support groups for pregnant women who have experienced pregnancy loss, and they report the same anxiety and fear. Despite seeing the baby's image on the sonogram screen, despite talking to their doctor, they still feel infertile. As Ellen Glazer says in her book *The Long Awaited Stork,* they are living in "no person's land," unable to emotionally or physically let go, and make the transition between infertility and pregnancy. Although initially elated at the news of a positive pregnancy test, they cannot celebrate their pregnancy like other women.[9]

As we spoke about in the introduction to this chapter, the old familiar voice of infertility does not die when the pregnancy test results are positive. The voice lives on, sometimes with more force than before, because now there is more at stake: a live baby inside you. So the voice tells you to be afraid, to not put too much stock in this pregnancy, to hold back and not bond with your baby. Why should you? Time after time, treatment after treatment, things have not worked out as planned. Many women describe feeling anxious during the first few months and then having periods when they feel safer, more calm. Others say they were fearful until they finally had their baby in their arms.

You will have to take your pregnancy one step at a time, hour by hour, or even minute by minute. If something feels physically uncomfortable or you are unsure about a sensation, you can always check with your doctor. Once your physician has allayed your fears, try to relax. If you still have trouble quieting negative thoughts, Aline Zoldbrod, a psychologist and author specializing in infertility, suggests using a *thought-stopping technique* to squelch the fear of pregnancy loss. When the negative thoughts invade, try screaming silently or out loud, "Stop!" "Some people even need to wear a rubber band around their wrist [loosely of course!] and snap it as they say, 'Stop.' "[10] Snapping and screaming will help you shift your gears and refocus to other more positive possibilities.

Also, try to surround yourself with supportive people, and accept that the trauma you have been through is real. The emotional transition from infertile to fertile will not happen overnight. During the times when you feel better, see if you can enjoy your pregnant state. You have waited a long time to get to the place you are in, and you deserve to enjoy it.

10. How Do I Stop Worrying about Miscarriage?

I've had four miscarriages this year, and now once again I'm pregnant. I'm still taking my temperature every morning before I get out of bed, even though it has been a month since my positive pregnancy test. I run to the bathroom all the time looking for blood. Whenever I feel the tiniest twinge, I start crying. I am afraid I'm going to lose this baby too. My husband thinks that I've really gone crazy. And I know he's right, but I can't seem to stop. What am I going to do?

Who wouldn't feel scared?

Zoldbrod, in her book *Men, Women and Infertility,* suggests that patients who find themselves anxious during their pregnancies utilize a mantra to stop their negative thoughts from taking over. Mantras are commonly used in prayer or meditation and help people to focus their thoughts. Zoldbrod encourages using the phrase, "So far, so good." As long as the patient has not heard any negative reports from her physician and is basing her fears on her past, she can confidently say, "So far, so good."[11]

Here are some other options:

1. Call your doctor if you are feeling something that is making you especially nervous. Some doctors will schedule frequent appointments, especially if you have had numerous miscarriages.
2. Try the stress management exercises mentioned in Appendix I, and if possible, use some of them on a daily basis.
3. Locate other pregnant women that will understand your concerns. Some RESOLVE chapters have established Pregnancy after Infertility groups; others have set up informal networks.
4. Take good care of yourself: eat well, exercise as much as medically advised, do things that make you feel good about yourself, and socialize with supportive family and friends.

11. I Don't Want to Complain about Complete Bed Rest, But . . .

As I went through my infertility, I swore that no one would ever hear me complain. Unlike the rest of the world, no matter what discomforts, pain, or inconvenience a pregnancy would cause me, I intended to smile through it. And I've really lived up to my promise. Even when I was vomiting everyday, I managed to keep going to work and basically continue my life as usual. But now I am confined to bed and all the added work for my husband—not to mention the fact that I'm not bringing any money home—has really been hard and is causing us both a lot of stress. But I can't tell anyone how badly I feel because I feel so guilty. I'm so lucky to be pregnant, how can I not be 100 percent grateful?

Candace Hurley, the founder of Sidelines (see their listing in Appendix II), a national help line for women on bed rest, said,

> After all I had been through, which was years of infertility and miscarriages, I now once again had to deal with the possibility of losing my baby. I was terrified and I was so lonely. When my doctor put me on complete bed rest for fourteen weeks, I felt as if I wasn't allowed to complain to anyone, but inside I knew I desperately needed support. When I did reach out, many people led me to believe that my disappointment and fear [were] wrong, that I was [being] ungrateful. But when I told my doctor how I was feeling, he suggested I call another one of his patients who had to be in bed during her pregnancy. That woman became my lifeline. She never once thought that my complaining and worries were unjustified. She knew [because] she had been there herself.[12]

You are not alone either. There are many women just like you, who are lying in their beds, pregnant, frightened, and lonely. Reach out to them. You will find that what you are experiencing is a normal reaction to an abnormal, frightening situation. Call Sidelines and learn that you can get the support you need.

12. How Can We Decide about Multifetal Pregnancy Reduction*?

After three unsuccessful IVF cycles my husband and I decided to try only one more cycle. Since it was our last try, we decided to put back all six fertilized embryos, instead of freezing half of them like we did during the other cycles. Finally after all these years we were getting our dream—I was pregnant! The euphoria came to an abrupt end last week when I found out I am carrying four fetuses. After the sonogram my doctor handed me a pamphlet on multifetal pregnancy reduction and said, "I urge you to consider it." And after reading the brochure I know why he suggested it. The brochure quoted all these statistics on the health of multiple-birth ba-

---

* *Multifetal pregnancy reduction,* also referred to as *selective reduction,* is a medical procedure used to reduce risks to mothers and babies in some instances of multiple gestation.[13]

bies and the mother who carries them. But there is also the risk of miscarriage after the reduction, so deciding to abort one or two could mean losing four. We don't know where to turn or what to do.

We are sorry that you have to deal with making this enormous decision, especially after the years you have spent struggling with your infertility. Considering all you have been through and what lies ahead, we urge you to go easy on yourselves and let go of the guilt you are carrying. Mary McKinney, Ph.D., who has done extensive research on multifetal pregnancy reduction, tells couples considering reducing their pregnancy, "Do not feel as if you're making this decision selfishly. You're not. Instead, this decision is about looking at the overall quality of your life; not just what you want for yourself, but what is best for your husband and your future children."[14] She also urges couples to think very carefully about the issue of privacy. In her study at Columbia Presbyterian Hospital in New York, she found that some couples who had gone through a reduction regretted having told close family and friends. Although they were appreciative of the help they received while they were in the midst of the crisis, afterwards they felt exposed and open to judgment. Many felt pressured to tell their children of their loss since others around them knew of their decision to reduce.

If at all possible, put your other responsibilities aside while making this decision. You will need all the time and energy you can gather. Rochelle Friedman, M.D., and Bonnie Gradstein, M.P.H., say in their book *Surviving Pregnancy Loss,* "Assimilating complex medical information and deciding what course of action to take can be difficult under any circumstance; at a time when you are in a state of shock and feeling overwhelmed it may be all you can do to think straight, much less make a critical decision in a short space of time."[15]

Maureen Boyle, executive director of Mothers of Supertwins (MOST; see listing in Appendix II), suggests that before making this decision you seek qualified responses to the following questions from both an obstetrician specializing in high-risk pregnancies (perinatologist) and a pediatrician who has experience with babies born prematurely (neonatologist):

- Will my pregnancy be managed differently if I had a reduction?
- If I had a reduction, would my pregnancy be considered high risk?
- What are the risks of prematurity?
- What are the risks of maternal complications?

- What measures can be taken during the pregnancy to prevent preterm delivery?
- How many reduced pregnancies has the obstetrician managed and what was the gestational outcome?
- What can be done during the pregnancy to reduce the complications to babies born early?
- How many sets of triplets (quadruplets or quintuplets) has the obstetrician delivered in the past year, and what was the average gestational outcome?*
- Will prolonged hospital stay for both you and your children be necessary during a multiple pregnancy? If so, what are the costs?[16]

Gathering information about the physical aspects of carrying multiples and the risks of multifetal pregnancy reduction will be a much less tedious task than finding information on the psychological aspects. One of the few studies done on the latter was conducted by McKinney. She and her colleagues interviewed forty-two women who had their pregnancies reduced as well as a control group of forty-four women who became pregnant through medical intervention but conceived only a single baby or twins and did not need reduction.

Most of the women coped well with the reduction when the outcome was successful births. However, the majority of women who went through the procedure found it sad and depressing to abort some of the fetuses. On the day of the procedure, all but one felt anxiety, 57 percent reported feeling guilty, and 69 percent felt sad or depressed. In a few cases, wives said their husbands found the procedure more stressful than they did.

In the study, eight women lost the entire pregnancy after the reduction and ten of the control group miscarried. All reported grief and mourning, and over two-thirds experienced symptoms that impaired their daily functioning for more than two weeks.

The women who underwent a reduction were no more likely than the control group of women to experience severe depression or longlasting psychiatric symptoms. When the pregnancy was successful, 15 percent of both multifetal pregnancy reduction patients and the control group reported symptoms indicative of depression at some point during the nine months prior to the interview. The au-

---

* According to Boyle, the national average gestation of women carrying multiples is 34 weeks for triplets (with no long-term problems associated with prematurity expected), 32 weeks for quadruplets (with an average 4-week hospital stay with some challenges while an inpatient but no long-term problems expected), and 30 weeks for quintuplets (with 98 percent of all babies born at this gestation surviving but some possibility of ongoing challenges associated with prematurity).

thors of the study concluded that when reduction is successful, it rarely leads to depression or other severe psychological problems. Most women felt they had made the best decisions for themselves and their families. In fact, over half the women said that infertility treatment and worrying about getting pregnant had been more stressful than the reduction. Only one woman who delivered healthy twins regretted her decision and wished that she had tried to carry triplets.[17]

You should note that this study neither addresses the long-term effects of multifetal pregnancy reduction nor compares the outcomes of reductions with the outcomes of those women who decided to carry their multiples to term.

RESOLVE and MOST will be able to put you in touch with women who have had a reduction and feel comfortable talking about their experience. MOST organization can give you information and support and will introduce you to families that have had a reduction and those with grand multiples, who can provide insight into the daily life of parenting. Talking with a professional trained to handle reproductive issues can help you deal with your intense emotions in a nonthreatening way and help both of you weigh the many sides of this complex but ultimately manageable decision. Because this is one of the most crucial times in your life, you should not have to deal with it alone.

IV

EPILOGUE

When infertility is over—when a baby is placed in your arms or a commitment to live child-free is solidified by the changes you make in your lifestyle—wondrous things happen.

For those who choose to parent, reentry into the world you temporarily left behind brings joy and happiness. Suddenly you are the one having the baby shower. You are the one standing in the baby isle in the supermarket, putting formula, diapers, and baby food in your cart. You are reading "Dr. Spock" and talking endlessly about diaper rash, colic, midnight feedings, pacifiers, and how to survive on no sleep. Suddenly all is right with the world: you have your baby, your story has changed; and your dream has come true.

For couples who choose a child-free lifestyle, the story is just as happy. You are free to pursue what you love most in life. Perhaps it is your work, helping others, nurturing a neice, or volunteering. Perhaps it's nurturing yourself creatively through writing, painting, singing, or another art form. Once again your relationship with your partner can grow. The pressure is off. It's the two of you for life, a commitment that feels good and solid. Because you've survived infertility as a couple, you can survive anything.

For all of you who have been through the experience of infertility, your own epilogue will be different. How comfortable you are with the choices you have made can only be judged with the passage of time.

The initial euphoria of resolution will eventually be replaced by the day-to-day realities of parenting or living child-free. And in the midst of this new life you will remember where you have been and who you were during that time. It may happen when you least expect it. You may hear a story about a cousin going through an IVF treatment, or you may see a woman breast-feeding her child in the mall, and suddenly it all comes back: the disappointments, the longings—how desperately you wanted to hold a baby, just like that woman in the mall.

The truth is, you will never forget. There will always be a place in your heart where your first baby—the one you would have conceived easily—would have lived. Seymour Fisher, in his book *Sexual Images of the Self,* calls this baby the "phantom fetus." As Aline Zoldbrod notes,

> One would presume that since the idea of being pregnant is so central to feminine identity, the average girl starts early to come to terms in fantasy with the

phantom fetus who is already a part of her body image. Fisher called this a potential "someone else who is or will be within me" state. . . . "By the time of adolescence and probably earlier the vast majority of girls have constructed images of [the] self as a potential creative container. The concept of being a protective womb is universally linked to womanhood."[1]

You now face both the loss of your identity as a fertile woman and the loss of that first baby. To know these losses for what they are is to keep them in perspective so you will not think they have anything to do with the children you now love or the child-free lifestyle you have chosen. You may always be infertile, but true resolution is about embracing the other parts of yourself. It is a process of sorting out, prioritizing, letting go, and accepting. It involves taking a good look at all you have learned, all you have accomplished, and all you have become: the stronger, wiser, more compassionate person who knows how to get through a major life crisis. As a woman who lost her mother to cancer told Hope Edelman in *Motherless Daughters*,

> "I've had people ask me, 'If some things could have happened differently in your life, what would they be?' . . . And I'd have to say there isn't anything I'd change. I'm sorry for different things that have happened, but I wouldn't have done it any other way. The losses are . . . so much a part of . . . my maturing, and . . . the person I am today. And I like who I am today. It stinks that these things had to happen to me, but I can make the decision to let them be a plus or a minus."[2]

And so it is too with infertility. You can decide how much of your life you are willing to hand over to this loss and how much of life you wish to retain. The epilogue to being infertile is not only about loss and endings. It is also about beginnings.

V

—

TREATING INFERTILITY

A Guide for Professionals

"It was the first time I had ever been to a therapist, I didn't know what to expect. I was really scared."

"My grandmother sees the need for therapy as sign of weakness. She has told me that when I am strong enough I will be able to handle my own problems."

"As soon as the therapist asked me what had been going on in my life I began to cry. Then I told her the whole story. It felt good to know that someone actually cared enough to ask. No one ever asked before."

"I had called about going into a support group, but by the time the therapist called me back the next day, I had changed my mind. It wasn't until a year later that I was able to call again, and really commit myself to going."

"The last thing I wanted to do was to be in a room full of women crying about their infertility. Believe me, my wife was enough. But the leader was good and I liked the other couples. To my surprise the group actually made me feel better in some ways."

"My support group saved my life. I couldn't believe I was actually sitting in a room full of women who felt the same way I did. Until that point I thought I was the only one who hated pregnant women."

These are the voices of men and women caught in a crisis. Infertility is a crisis so intense and so painful, it has the power to transform one's very core. Beliefs, dreams, and identity shift forever in the wake of this experience. Seeking the help of a professional can be the first step in finding the support, understanding, and validation needed during this difficult and uncertain time.

The therapeutic environment offers a safe haven to talk, vent, and deal with the roller coaster of emotions that take place during each menstrual cycle. Therapy is the one place clients can both hold on to and let go of their feelings, where they can come to terms with the instability infertility has wreaked on their lives and find the strength and hope necessary to move beyond the crisis.

What does the therapist need to know about the infertile client in order to meet these needs? How does the professional approach this relationship? What is a "normal" reaction to the crisis of infertility, and how is treating the infertility patient different from treating other clients in your practice? These questions are the focus of this chapter. In addition to presenting various treatment approaches and ways to help the infertile individual, couple, and group deal with this crisis, we found a number of issues that therapists will want to be aware of. We offer the following points of information and guidelines in order to paint as complete a picture as possible of the psychotherapeutic treatment of infertility:*

VALIDATION

There is nothing more important to an infertility client than to know that their feelings are valid, and that they are not "crazy." Sit with almost any group of infertility clients and you will hear them say over and over again, "I know this is crazy but . . ." or "I want to tell my doctor this, but I'm afraid he'll think I'm crazy," or most often, "My husband thinks I'm crazy." Therapists can help their clients by challenging these perceptions and offering other ways for clients to view their thoughts and feelings.

HOPE

After validation, the second most important thing therapists can offer their clients is hope. Realistic yet positive support can stay with clients during their darkest hours. It is important to tell patients that infertility is a temporary crisis. If they want to become parents, they will find a way. Resolution eventually occurs, and with it will come a sense of peace.

FLEXIBILITY IN FEES AND SCHEDULING

For those therapists who work with infertility patients, flexibility in both scheduling and fee practices can be a key factor in the success of the relationship. According

---

* In writing this chapter we drew on our many years of experience working with infertility patients as well as the most current literature regarding the psychotherapeutic treatment of this population. We also asked a respected group of therapists to write summaries for us of their experiences and give their recommendations for working with infertility patients. Here and elsewhere we have quoted from the papers they submitted to us. A list of the contributors and their professional affiliations is given at the end of Part V.

to Randi Guggenheimer, R.N., C.S.W., the disruptive nature of infertility leaves its mark on the therapeutic relationship as cancellations and schedule changes become both frequent and necessary. Whether it is a sonogram, a blood test, an insemination, or even an IVF transfer, both the therapist and client are at the mercy of the patient's reproductive cycle. In light of this, clients need to be able to cancel appointments without the risk of being labeled resistant or inconsiderate. Policies that monetarily penalize clients for missed appointments are incompatible with the treatment of infertility patients.

Clients undergoing infertility treatment may also need more flexibility from the therapist with regard to their fees. Costs for medical treatment, often not covered by insurance, can run into the thousands of dollars (over $9,000 for an average IVF cycle, for example), leaving some individuals or couples unable to pay for therapy. The therapist needs to recognize that making medical treatment for infertility a priority over almost anything else in the client's life is appropriate at this time. Therefore, clients asking for a reduced fee should not be automatically viewed as being resistant to beginning or continuing therapy.[1]

When the Therapist Is *Not* Infertile

Believing that only another infertile individual can truly understand their experience, most infertile clients prefer knowing that their therapist has shared a similar fate. Although being infertile is not a prerequisite for working successfully with infertility clients, understanding that the issue of identification is very pronounced for them is.

Most infertility patients will come into the therapist's office already feeling cut off from other members of their gender. Feeling misunderstood and alone in the outside world, many seek support and understanding from "one who knows." Clients who have to explain the medical terminology and treatment information to the therapist may believe (albeit incorrectly) that their feelings also are not being understood. Therefore, it is important for the fertile therapist to be prepared by becoming knowledgeable about testing, treatments, and options in family building. "Therapists may also reveal their sensitivity to the many feelings surrounding infertility by selectively sharing, from their own lives, incidents which brought up for them comparable feelings of being out of control, of sadness, loss, anger, or anxiety. Good therapists can use their own experiences to touch their clients."[2]

WHEN THE THERAPIST *IS* INFERTILE

The therapist who has experienced infertility may seem like a godsend to the infertile client. There is no question that those with a personal history of infertility are able to understand both the medical and emotional issues from the inside.

However, therapeutically, such qualifications offer the client no assurances of a successful alliance. In fact, overidentification with a client can be as much of a hindrance to the therapeutic process as underidentification. Therefore, the therapist who has experienced infertility will want to be extremely clear about his or her own issues to avoid any unnecessary countertransference.

For one therapist who found resolution and happiness through adoption, working with clients exploring child-free options was difficult.

> When I first adopted my daughter, I was so happy being a mother, I could not understand why anyone would reject the idea of adoption. Sometimes I felt angry when I heard my clients say that if they couldn't give birth to a baby, they would rather live without children. It didn't make sense to me since they had spent so many years trying to become a parent. But the further I got away from my own infertility issues, the easier it was for me to see child-free living as a viable option. I know now I am better equipped to help people make a clear choice.

Being watchful of such issues and working to move through them offers both client and therapist opportunities for understanding and growth.

DIAGNOSIS

The emotional reactions to infertility might seem severe in presentation, yet typically they fall within the normal and expected range of responses. Sonia Hieger, C.S.W., B.C.D., a therapist specializing in infertility, writes:

> I have come to be able to clearly see the profound helplessness that the client experiences, the feeling of being stuck with one's life at a standstill. As a result, every client that I see for infertility is in a depression, which is the "normal" reaction to helplessness, to the feeling of impotency in one's life. Every client is also anxious, some keeping it contained through various and unique coping mechanisms. The men often do it through work, through sports, and through denial. The women may do it through trying to focus on their jobs, through food, through shopping, and possibly escaping through sleep.[3]

Therefore, clients who seek the help of a professional in their search for answers do not do so as a reaction to some form of mental illness, but rather as an ongoing process of health. Providers of health insurance, however, demand that therapists provide a diagnosis for treatment. The diagnoses in the DSM IV that seem to give the closest fit are "adjustment disorder with mixed anxiety and depressed mood" (309.28) and "posttraumatic stress disorder" (309.81).[4] The nonorganic nature of these diagnoses and the recognition that the health of the person has been challenged by circumstances beyond his or her control draw us most strongly to these diagnoses.

Patient or Client?

Those who are infertile are "infertility clients," not "mental health patients." Labeling clients as "patients" implies a lack of health or illness, neither of which hold true for the vast majority of infertile individuals we encounter. This is why we use the term "patients" only when referring to their medical status and "clients" when referring to their status as consumers of mental health services.

Seeing Clearly

It is important to help infertility clients see that it is the limitations of medical science and the body's physiology that are causing their infertility and not something they are doing wrong. Treatment providers often communicate varying messages of blame to infertile women. This is especially true for a woman undergoing IVF, who after the transfer procedure returns home with fertilized eggs in her body. "Feeling" pregnant, she anxiously waits for confirmation. If the pregnancy test comes back negative or if she miscarries, the physician who is not careful may leave the patient feeling that it was her fault. Traditionally, the assumption has been that the treatment is a success once the transfer of fertilized eggs has been completed. This can be seen in the reporting of statistics that give only transfer rates and do not include actual live birth rates. Viewing these statistics as truth, a woman who miscarries may be under the impression that her experience is atypical or that she did something wrong since she was unable to carry those embryos to term. Women need to be told outright by all the professionals who work with them—doctors, nurses, and therapists—that when a procedure does not work, it is not her failure but rather the treatment that failed. Women must be allowed to see that it is technology that is limited, thus reducing the risk of self-blame and incrimination.

WHO THE GATEKEEPERS ARE

Finally, there are some questions every therapist working in the IVF clinic or reproductive endocrinologist's office should consider:

- Does the therapist have the right to decide who should be allowed medical treatment and who should be denied? For example, should the infertility patient who presents with severe depression be allowed to continue medical treatment for infertility? How about women who are alcoholic, obese, abused, or who suffer from phobias or panic attacks? Does anyone stop fertile couples from reproducing?
- What are the obligations around confidentiality? Does the therapist confide in the nurses and doctors, or does she keep confidential what her client has told her?
- Whose best interest will the therapist look after? Is it in the best interest of the physicians who own the clinic that their patients continue treatment?

Most importantly, the therapist in the physician's office can offer education and advocacy to clients by helping them explore all their options and by informing them of the realities and implications of various medical procedures.

1. When Is It Appropriate to Encourage Grief Work?

I have a client who has been dealing with infertility for four years. She's been through three IVF cycles and two miscarriages and is finally ready to end her struggle with medical treatment and move on to adoption. Although she is relieved about ending treatment and joyous about the prospect of becoming a parent, I sense she is conflicted about leaving all medical treatment behind. I believe her unspoken hesitancy stems from her unresolved grief over the many losses she has suffered. However, she does not seem ready to truly mourn, especially when it concerns the loss of her pregnancies, future pregnancy, or a genetically related child. When is the appropriate time to encourage an infertile client to begin grief work? What specific exercises or rituals are helpful in encouraging grief work?

As a woman moves from one unsuccessful treatment to the next, she will experience many losses. If this were a perfect world, each of these losses would be validated and mourned. The body would have time to move back to its center, and the woman would be able to move on to the next cycle with new-found strength and the knowledge that support will always be there for her. But for most women, the arrival of her period and the emotional devastation accompanying it are quickly replaced by renewed hope and the possibilities of a new cycle. Mourning, if it takes place at all, is never completed.

For therapists the challenge is in finding a balance between helping their clients grieve each of these losses and supporting the clients' wishes to move quickly, with hope and optimism, to the next cycle. Ideally, grieving should be encouraged whenever time allows and the client shows a readiness to do so. However, often these opportunities are few within the confines of the twenty-eight-day menstrual cycle. The client who leaves your office on a Thursday and finds her period on Friday will, by the time you see her again, be gearing up for the rigors of her next cycle. To encourage mourning at this point would be both counterproductive and out of synch with the realities of her life. Therefore, many therapists have found that infertility patients often leave medical treatment with a multitude of unresolved loss issues. This is especially true when miscarriages, ectopic pregnancies, or early infant death are a part of their history.

Often the decision to end medical treatment signals the first opportunity for therapists to help their clients begin the grieving process. However, our experience tells us that the true letting go of the complex losses associated with infertility cannot be fully realized until after the client has moved on to the next life stage. Whether this means the arrival of biological or adopted children, or a commitment to a child-free lifestyle, infertile clients must have something new to hold on to before letting go of dreams that sustained them for so long.

One approach often used to help clients face this unresolved grief is Gestalt therapy:

> By using a powerful phenomenological methodology, the Gestalt therapist works in the present centeredness of the ongoing therapeutic relationship. Through skillful observation of what is present (language and body cues, client's contact with herself and the therapist), the therapist learns much about the client's dynamics. Gestalt theory of holism recognizes that the body, mind, and emotions are so interrelated that one does not function separately of the other two. And the therapist knows that the intrinsic will to survive and thrive requires that what remains unfinished (unexpressed emotions, trauma) be pushed forward to be actualized.[5]

According to Joyce Magid, C.S.W., working with loss requires therapists using a
Gestalt approach to be

> keenly aware of the many layers of the client's psyche. They must be able and
> willing to guide the client through the intense grieving and bear the client's pain.
> They must be able to offer support while helping the client explore the recesses
> of herself and hear the sound of her own wailing. The therapist must be
> grounded in the belief that by the client's experience, as well as her resistances,
> she can move through the letting-go process with sanity, self awareness, support,
> and a real connection to her real experience.

With the help of the Gestalt therapist, the client is able to explore " 'behind and
below' the surface, and move gently, and with the client's permission, into the less
accessible terrain of the emotions, the body and the soul." Unresolved beliefs and
issues can then rise to the surface allowing the client to come face to face with herself and what infertility is for her.

> For one woman, her belief about never getting what she wants will be con-
> firmed. For another, her intrinsic differentness, unworthiness, and emptiness are
> proven. A twenty-nine-year-old man will come to face his sense of his manhood.
> A thirty-eight-year-old woman faces the grief of a secret teenage pregnancy. A
> young woman, who dreamed of pregnancy as long as she remembers, finds her-
> self disappearing before her eyes. Another who has long despised her body, ex-
> periences its ultimate betrayal.
>
> It is in this landscape that the Gestalt therapist uncovers the volcanoes of
> rage, the deep underground pools of tears, the mirrors of illusions, the scarred
> fields of traumas and the endless miracles of resilient hopes and dreams. The
> Gestalt therapist engages in the sacred work of healing by taking the hand of the
> wounded client and leading her/him lovingly and skillfully through the difficult
> journey.

Piece by piece as the client retrieves her original authentic self, she begins to fully
experience the richness of her life. For the first time she is able to acknowledge
with respect and appreciation the phrase "I am infertile." By embracing her experiences, courage, tenacity, pain, loss, regrets, and victories, she allows herself her true
emotions. When the words "I am infertile" no longer are her total identity but only
one aspect of it, which recedes into the background of herself as the poet, the
friend, the teacher, the lawyer, the mother, she is truly healing the deepest of her
wounds.

When the client is ready, the time will come for a symbolic yet tangible way to express most fully the meaning these losses have held for her. She will need a ceremonial way to say goodbye to all that preceded that day.

> Because there are no rituals with which to grieve unborn children in our culture, encouraging the client to work this through by accepting and validating her feelings can enable her to go forward with her grief. This can be done by planting a tree or bush in the couple's backyard or someplace else where they feel comfortable, releasing balloons into the air, or burying other symbols of their grief.
>
> In the case of miscarriage, the couple can bury anything related to the baby: pictures of sonograms, positive pregnancy tests, hospital bracelets, pictures of the baby as well as the baby. The couple can then choose to have a service commemorating their child. While some clients may feel uncomfortable with this idea, those who do partake in these ceremonies report feeling a sense of relief that they have now laid their baby to rest. And some, feel that they have laid the idea of a biological child to rest.[6]

Magid describes one such journey taken by a client who, after many years of losses, was able to let go and say goodbye to all the unborn babies she had held inside her for so long:

> They silently stood in the yard, their bare feet buried in the moist summer earth. Two shopping bags of charts rested in the shadows of the shade trees. The birds, their fluttering quieted, settled on the branches above. The Dalmation ceased his search for the elusive squirrel and found his place at the base of the oak tree. They gathered together—the client, the therapist, and nature's witnesses—to put to rest ten years of suffering, raging, longing, denying. It was time, after a courageous therapeutic journey, to metaphorically bury years of menstrual cycle monitoring charts, an ectopic pregnancy, and dreams of a pregnancy and a birth child. It was time to say farewell to the birth child who would never be, who would never live to be held by this mother. It was time to honor her grieving, her unfulfilled dreams, and her valiant fight.
>
> She took the lighted match from the therapist, her guide through the journey, and carefully caught the bottom right corner of the chart that rested on top of the pile. She watched as the fire spread through the charts. She held another match to the next pile, and the next, until all that remained was a hill of ashes.
>
> She dug a hole in the earth and shoveled the ashes into the hole. Then she placed the small yellow rattle and the tiny doll, once bought for the baby who never lived, on top of the soft ashes. Her tears moistened the contents as she cov-

ered the burial site with the remaining earth. She placed a small stone on the site and stood for several moments in a final farewell. She took her therapist's hand, and together they walked from the memorial into the light of the summer sun.[7]

Although for this woman, as with all infertility patients, there will be many scars and monthly reminders of the pain suffered, it must also be remembered that there is always life after infertility. And it is the therapist who holds for the client "the possibility and hope that life is good, that she is alive and well and that she can again have herself and her life—richly, choicefully and creatively."[8]

2. What Therapeutic Methods Are Useful in Counseling the Infertile Couple?

For the past year I have been working with an infertile couple. They basically have a good marriage, except when it comes to issues surrounding their infertility. Their biggest problem is that they are always fighting over what course of treatment they should follow. First he wanted inseminations and she wanted IVF. They decided on three cycles of each. Then she wanted to adopt and he said *one* more cycle of IVF. So they did one more cycle and now she's talking donor sperm and he is talking adoption. Is this constant struggle common among infertile couples? What if any issues are typical for this population, and what therapeutic techniques are helpful in counseling them?

Infertile couples come into the therapist's office in the middle of a major life crisis. They are struck, usually early on in their marriage, with a problem that touches them socially, emotionally, physically, and financially. Scared about the state of their relationship, anxious about the outcome of medical treatment and the possible loss of their fertility and a biological child, and often disagreeing over what course of treatment to follow, they look to the therapist for help. The therapist becomes the guide, illuminating a path toward the answers they seek, and finding ways to help them come to terms with this crisis.

Therapists can work within various treatment modalities and use a myriad of techniques and exercises to create support, understanding, and validation for their clients. The following tools have proven to be highly successful in working with infertile couples.

GENOGRAMS

Nancy Newman, M.S.W., believes that before the therapist can begin to help the couple gain the insight needed to make decisions and move on in the resolution process, it is important to take into account that infertile couples often experience a plethora of involvements from outside systems, be they medical, social, or familial.* She suggests that the therapist use a multigenerational, family-of-origin approach in order to see clearly how these systems as well as unresolved family conflicts might influence clients' perceptions of themselves as well as the eventual outcomes of their infertility. She encourages therapists to use a genogram† during initial visits. By mapping out the key players in the client's life and obtaining a developmental and functional history of the family, you will be able to obtain answers to crucial questions such as:

1. Are your client's losses around infertility complicated by other losses within the family of origin or previous generation?
2. What is the meaning of family, and how does that influence your client's response to his or her infertility? (For example, does the client's family believe that a person does not become an adult until he or she becomes a parent?)
3. Is your client willing to go to any length to have a family in order to make up for prior family losses? (Some couples cannot let go of their grief. No matter how many therapists they see or how many support groups they join, they are unable to come to grips with their loss. What emerges time and again is the grief around infertility goes unresolved because of a prior loss(es), for example, around a parent's death, a miscarriage, or some other early childhood trauma.[9]

---

* Newman believes that the professional (nurse, physician, or mental health care provider) who works with infertile couples needs to examine his or her own emotional, ethical, and religious beliefs to see whether he or she is likely to influence the couple's personal decision-making process. What are the therapist's feelings about high-tech treatment options, adoption, child-free living, and so on? Since many who work in the field have experienced infertility themselves, it is important to know which issues will trigger reactivity and to reduce that as much as possible.

† Monica McGoldrick and Randy Gerson's book *Genograms and Family Assessment* (W. W. Norton and Co., New York, 1986) provides a good overview on the use of genograms.

GENDER-RELATED ISSUES AND "THE COUPLES DIALOGUE"

The woman, because of her anatomy, is usually more involved with the medical system than her husband, regardless of whether the infertility is caused by the male, the female, a combination, or remains unexplained. The female therefore often focuses her attention on finding the "right" treatment, which makes her more susceptible to self blame and guilt. The man, on the other hand, experiences infertility "less physically and more abstractly." He involves himself with work and taking care of "things." It can be difficult to help him move past the role of caretaker. If the man is unable to shift his position, his partner may feel he is not dealing with his own pain regarding the infertility. She may therefore feel unsupported, leading to emotional distancing between the partners.[10]

To address this distancing, Ira Kalina, Ph.D., director of Couple Works, a center for marital therapy on Long Island, believes in a threefold approach to therapy. First, the therapist serves as an advocate for the marriage and finding the good in what the couple are trying to do with each other. This encourages an atmosphere of trust, empathy, and safety that will enable the couple to gradually bring up what matters most to them about their shared lives and the impact infertility has had on their relationship. Second, the therapist teaches them to notice repetitive negative patterns and helps them develop skills so they can choose successful alternatives. Third, the therapist teaches, models, and practices these alternatives in the working crucible of the psychotherapist's office.[11]

Since all three of these goals require the couple to communicate effectively, Kalina teaches his clients "The Couple's Dialogue,"* a framework for communication that employs the following guidelines:

1. Partners learn to listen and mirror one another.
2. Partners take responsibility for feelings by using "I" statements. They also learn to empathize with and validate their partner through a deeper understanding of the partner's life history and struggles.
3. Each partner learns to define and clearly communicate his or her wants, needs, and desires; couples are then better prepared to talk about issues no matter how difficult or threatening the subject.[12]

For more details of this process, see Chapter 3.

---

* The theory of Imago Relationship Therapy, in which The Couple's Dialogue is an integral component, was developed by Hendrix in 1979.

DECISION MAKING

Quite often a stumbling block to resolving infertility is the inability of couples to agree on what course of treatment to pursue. Author and infertility specialist Linda Salzar, L.C.S.W., A.C.S.W., asks her clients to make lists of the specific treatments they are contemplating. She asks them to describe the pros and cons of each treatment and to assign each a number from 1 to 10. The partners compare their lists and discuss the similarities and differences.

She also encourages her clients to read books about resolution options that express a variety of viewpoints. This challenges their belief systems and opens the door to discussions they otherwise might have been reluctant to bring up with one another.[13]

SEX AND INFERTILITY

It is important for psychotherapists to be aware that infertility has most likely adversely affected if not temporarily ended the couple's sexual relationship. "Lovemaking becomes work, effort, sometimes a stressful chore that needs to be 'accomplished' within a certain number of hours. After several years of 'clinical sex,' either performed at home or in the doctor's office through inseminations, or even in a petri dish, most couples have forgotten that lovemaking is about desire and attraction."[14] The couple might even avoid the sexual act altogether because it reminds them of their failure to conceive as well as the lack of the child they want so desperately. Therapists can best help these couples by suggesting ways to "get away" from their infertility both physically and mentally. A full discussion of suggestions on how to do this is provided in Chapter 1.

LOSS OF THE DREAM CHILD

One of the greatest losses faced by infertile couples is the loss of the child they had dreamed of creating together. It is also one of the most difficult losses to grieve because "no one helps them to acknowledge that their grief is real. There is no baby. If someone is there and then dies, every one can support the grieving person. How does one get support for the loss of someone who was never there?" This is the critical role of the therapist. By helping couples to "see" the child that will never be, therapists help their clients to feel their grief and acknowledge their pain. The following questions can help to make the loss more real for couples.

· Will your unborn child be a boy or girl?
· What hair and eye color will the child have?
· Will the child look like you or your husband or a combination of both?
· Whose talents will he or she have?
· Whose personality traits will the child have?[15]

Once the grief and sorrow are brought to the surface, the therapist can suggest a healing ritual that honors their experience of infertility or pregnancy loss. (Different rituals are described elsewhere in this chapter as well as in Chapter 8.) The sharing and planning of the ritual can bring a sense of renewal to the relationship and can also be the first opportunity the couple has to reconnect and find their way back to one another.[16] (See question 1 for a more thorough discussion of grief work with infertile couples.) And finding their way back to one another during this crisis carves the path not only to the resolution of their infertility but to their future as well. The therapist who works with infertile couples has the unique opportunity of guiding their clients through the medical, emotional, social, and financial crises of infertility, all the while helping them design a blueprint for a lifetime of solid crisis management skills.

3. What Should I Know about Leading an Infertility Support Group?

I am a social worker in the obstetrics and gynecology department for a large metropolitan hospital. Recently the reproductive endocrinologists approached me about running a support group for their patients. Although I have worked with infertile individuals and couples before, I have never conducted a group with them. What specific exercises have you found to be best suited for this group?

The following information will help you establish a secure atmosphere and build a solid foundation for leading support groups for infertility patients.

BUILDING TRUST: SETTING THE PARAMETERS OF THE GROUP

By setting the parameters right from the start, the group leader can provide a safe shelter for self-exploration and decision making. We recommend that groups be time-limited—between ten and fourteen weeks—and run for one and a half to two hours once a week. Members should be told that more sessions can be added if requested. Knowing the time boundaries of the group can help members set both short- and long-term goals. We also recommend not allowing new members to join the group after the second week. Further, we suggest keeping the groups homogeneous, limiting the composition to only primary or secondary infertility patients.

The location is also important. If at all possible, arrange for the group to meet outside a medical setting. A more neutral location can aid in promoting an environment in which members feel they can openly discuss their thoughts and feelings about their physician and his or her staff, treatment plans, financial demands, and so forth. Members need to know that their concerns are held in strict confidence by the leader and other members. The groups that take place within a physician's office or in a clinic setting traditionally have not offered members such trust.

Another issue that affects trust in the group process, and is hotly debated among professionals, is what happens when a group member gets pregnant. Those practitioners who argue for keeping pregnant women in the group believe that every infertile person must confront and deal with pregnancy in their daily lives and can work through their issues within the secure setting of the support group. They also argue that the women who achieve pregnancy continue to need the support lent to them by the other group members.

We feel differently. It has been our experience that when pregnant and infertile women are kept in groups together, no one's needs get met. Even though the pregnant woman's infertile feelings do not vanish after receiving a positive result on a pregnancy test, she will want to talk openly and freely about her bodily changes and the reactions of others. The pregnant woman needs to have a place to talk about her joy and excitement as well as her fear of loss, especially if she has had prior miscarriages. Infertile women may want to be supportive of the pregnant woman, but typically cannot help feeling jealous and angry, and subsequently guilty for having these feelings. They feel they need to hold themselves back from expressing their resentment toward the fertile world in the presence of the pregnant group member and cannot bear to hear about her problems—problems that they long to have.

Our solution to providing support to these two groups—the still infertile and the newly pregnant—has been to separate them. It is important, however, that this decision be made by the leader of the group and not by the group members themselves. The infertility support group goes on and alternative arrangements are made for the pregnant women, such as private counseling or a separate support group. The Long Island chapter of RESOLVE established a "pregnancy after infertility network," whereby pregnant members are able to contact each other for support and if needed can call a professional support group leader for advice.

GROUP INTERVENTIONS AND TECHNIQUES

Setting Goals[17] Once the parameters around the group are established, the group process begins to unfold. During the first session the leader can ask the members to establish the goals they have for themselves. By verbalizing their intentions, the members can stay somewhat focused on meeting their objectives over the course of the group. Most will talk about wanting to gain more control over their medical treatment; making decisions; dealing with their fertile family, friends, and co-workers; understanding their spouse's reaction to the problem; and developing general coping skills.

As the members of the group explore their feelings and experiences, they begin to learn from one another. Even when they are at different stages of the infertility process, the sharing of information, referrals, and feedback can be valuable. The leader can highlight the different approaches members take to similar situations and encourage further exploration of options. Armed with new skills and the feeling that decisions will be supported by the group, members are better able to negotiate uncomfortable situations.

Stress Management We have mentioned the value of stress management throughout the book and discussed its application to individual clients in this chapter. We also believe stress management should be incorporated into every support group as a means of coping with the crisis of infertility. We try to close each group with a ten- to twenty-minute relaxation exercise that typically includes deep breathing and guided imagery. This not only teaches members the skills they need to practice stress management techniques at home, but allows them to leave the session open and relaxed. (For specific techniques see Appendix I.)

Buddy System The buddy system, as introduced to us by Alice Domar, Ph.D., is a formalized vehicle for supporting members outside of meetings. Group participants are asked to make contact with at least one other group member during the week. In the groups we run, we randomly choose partners by picking and matching names from a hat during the first or second meeting. The buddies then trade phone numbers and are asked to talk to one another at least once before the next meeting. If there is an odd number of group members, a buddy triangle is established in which three partners are asked to talk during the week.

The buddy system addresses two of the main objectives of the infertility support group: counteracting isolation, and encouraging nurturing and caring relationships. It also speeds up the bonding among group members, a process that can otherwise take three to six weeks.

New and Good Activity   Each week, group members are asked to do something good for themselves by participating in an activity they believe will help them get through a difficult treatment or promote a healthful change in their lives. Most members report such activities as going for a walk, listening to music, taking a long bath, calling a friend they have not spoken with recently, and buying their favorite dessert after a particularly difficult doctor's visit. The New and Good Activity report, although difficult for some members in the beginning, encourages self-nurturing during this stressful time.

Another way to approach the New and Good Activity is to ask members to think and report on something that happened to them during the last week that felt new and good. Since infertility promotes negative thinking patterns, encouraging members to think of something good advances a more positive outlook.

You can use the New and Good Activity report as an opening or closing for the group. Both work equally as well. Be aware of those members who are not completing the New and Good Activity assignment; we have found an underlying depression in women who continually make excuses for not accomplishing this activity.

Journal Keeping   Group members are asked to keep infertility journals (see Appendix I). Some women will use the journal simply to keep track of their cycles and the emotional highs and lows as these relate to menstruation and medical treatments. Keeping records helps clients anticipate when a new treatment will begin and helps them to schedule their lives accordingly.

Clients are also encouraged to use their journals as an emotional outlet. Writing can be especially helpful for those who tend to be excessively anxious or obsessive or who have trouble expressing their feelings face to face.[18]

Externalization of the Infertility   Some individuals or couples will enter a support group feeling totally engulfed by their infertility. Others will be in the midst of "fighting the takeover." Externalization (as opposed to internalization) is a powerful technique, used by narrative therapists, that offers group members a way of separating their infertility problem from their identity. To externalize the infertility, try these techniques:

1. *Ask Clients to Bring Something to the Group that Represents Their Infertility*
   In deciding what objects to bring, the client is taking the infertility from the inside to the outside and placing its essence on something other than themselves. Some clients bring in wedding pictures and talk about their squelched dreams; others bring in objects relating to superstitions and magical thinking. Ask each member to describe the meaning of the object and what feeling it elicits.

2. *Ask Clients to Draw a Pie Chart*   Have group members draw a circle, divide it into pieces (like a pie), and label the pieces to represent the different parts of themselves. This exercise gives clients a visual portrayal of how much or how little of their identity they have "given up" to infertility. (See Chapter 1 for a description and samples of pie charts.) If the infertile-part slice is large, this acknowledges both the suffering that has taken place as well as the extent to which other parts of the person have been compromised by the problem. It also provides opportunities for clients to make choices as to how much power they will continue to give to infertility.

   Client's charts change depending on the treatment they are in and the day of their menstrual cycle they are on. For instance, if a member is waiting to hear about the outcome of an IVF cycle, the infertile part of her will be portrayed as large. However, if she has decided to take a break from treatment, or is in the beginning of a new menstrual cycle, she will most likely see the other parts of herself as larger than her infertility.

3. *Talk to the Group as If the Infertility Were a Person with an Identity and Will of Its Own*   To dramatize the personification, place an empty chair in the middle of the room and ask the members to imagine that *Infertility is sitting in the room with them.* You can pose questions to the group such as "What are the words Infertility whispers in your ear? How long has Infertility been in your life? in your bedroom? in your office?" And so on.

   Once the clients get a mental picture of Infertility, ask them to *write a letter* to the image. This can either be done during the meeting itself or assigned as homework. (We like to assign the letter as a homework project since the client can spend more time fantasizing about who Infertility is and what he or she would say to it.) Then ask the members to volunteer to read their letters to the group. (Generally every group member will participate.) This is usually a very insightful session as the members share the intense meanings they have given to the experience of infertility. It has also been the turning point for many group members as they suddenly became less willing to allow the infertility to take over their lives.

Art Therapy[19]   Clients can explore their conflicts, thoughts, and feelings about infertility through the use of art therapy.★ Much like the images that arise in dreams, the symbols that come from this type of therapy arrive on the blank page from the unconscious.

Art therapist Sheryl Stern suggests one such technique whereby members are given pieces of white paper and asked to note for themselves the word that enters their minds when they think of infertility. The leader then asks someone to volunteer to share his or her word with the group. If the other members agree that the word represents a common truth, all are asked to draw, with colored markers or pencils, the image this word conjures up. For example, a word commonly mentioned is "barren." One member might depict "barren" as an empty house. Another might mark the letter X on the page. The leader and group participants can then explore what these symbols represent. Does the empty house mean there is no child to fill it? Does the letter X mean a crossing out of who the client believes she is or what the experience infertility has done to her?

To further increase the members' connections with one another, the process is repeated until each person has shared the word that came to mind, the group has depicted what each stated word means, and all have shown their drawings to one another. The group gets a strong sense of camaraderie as they produce a quilt of images sewn together by shared thoughts and feelings.

As the support group leader, you can incorporate any or all of these techniques as long as you keep in mind that there are always two underlying goals of the group: to promote self-insight and growth, and to create a community of support. The clients we have known who have participated in infertility support groups almost always develop new social and emotionally supportive networks, sometimes even creating friendships that can last a lifetime.

4. Should I Use Cognitive Therapy or Antianxiety Medication?

I have been seeing a client for six months who came into therapy because she was having difficulty at work. She was making good use of the therapy and had

---

★ Clients who participate in art therapy need not have art experience or talent and should not be judged on their creativity.

come to terms with most of her issues concerning her boss, work schedule, and so forth. However, at the same time her problems at work had begun, she had entered medical treatment for infertility. For the past year and a half, she has been taking fertility drugs and having artificial inseminations using her husband's sperm.

Over the past two months, I have seen her grow increasingly anxious, depressed, and at times almost obsessed with getting pregnant. She can't focus on much else in her sessions. She speaks of being constantly upset, just not feeling like herself. And this anxiety and depression are becoming socially debilitating. She is having trouble being in the company of pregnant co-workers, family, and friends; most of the time she seeks isolation. She speaks openly of anger and cannot control her resentment.

I am unsure how to proceed with her. I would like to use some cognitive therapy approaches, but my supervision group feels this client might be helped by antianxiety medication. Are there any contraindications for using antianxiety medication for women trying to conceive? If I decide on a more cognitive approach, which methods work best with infertile clients?

Before we answer your questions regarding drug treatments and cognitive therapy, some comments on the profile you offer of your client are appropriate. Her increasing anxiety, depression, obsessive thoughts, and even her withdrawal from social gatherings involving pregnant women—all seem to be within the normal range of reactions to the crisis of infertility. People typically react to infertility as they would to any life crisis. Their focus becomes very narrow; all attention is paid to getting through each day, each test, and each treatment. To others this may seem obsessive, but to your client it feels like a matter of life and death for the baby she longs to carry.

Your client is at the point where she has been trying the same treatment for a very long time. She now faces new and perhaps more potent drugs; higher-tech and more invasive, time-consuming, and expensive procedures; as well as the ever-present, increasing possibility of never conceiving. Under these circumstances, *not* having episodes of depression and anxiety would seem pathological. Your client's anger and her choice to isolate herself from pregnant women is actually a healthy response to situations that have become too painful. In counseling we encourage infertile women to do whatever is necessary to make themselves comfortable during this time in their lives, even if it means dissociating from family and friends. Your client, like all the other infertile women we have seen, will return to her family and friends when she is better able to cope with her own feelings.

Anger is another example of a healthy response to a client's infertility and is a necessary component of the healing process. As her therapist, you must walk that fine line between validating these angry feelings and helping her attend to the accuracy of her thoughts. Acknowledging the differences between thoughts and feelings is an integral part of cognitive therapy.

Dominic Candido, Ph.D., and Teresa Candido, C.S.W., of the Long Island (N.Y.) Center for Cognitive Therapy, elaborate on the principles of cognitive therapy and its use in treating infertility clients:[20]

Developed by Aaron Beck, M.D., University of Pennsylvania, and other researchers such as Albert Ellis, Ph.D., at the Institute for Rational Emotive Therapy, cognitive therapy strategies for infertile individuals and couples can be used in a variety of contexts and settings. The strategies are appropriate at all stages of infertility, from consideration of initiation of procedures through symptoms which recur years after significant reproductive events have taken place. The main premise of cognitive therapy is that thought influences emotion. The extent to which individuals see themselves in a clear and accurate fashion determines their ability to cope with problems.

Cognitive therapy rests on two basic principles that, in our experience, determine the extent to which the therapy will be helpful in assisting persons and couples with problems of infertility: collaborative empiricism and Socratic questioning. Collaborative empiricism refers to the extent to which the therapist and patient(s) work together to uncover the truth in their world. It is the basis upon which goals are made, clinical procedures are contracted, and the therapeutic alliance is formed. Socratic questioning is a moment-to-moment intervention used by the therapist to teach the ability to question one's own experience and to elicit knowledge from the client. Truth is assumed to be known by the infertility client. The therapist's task is to elicit this truth from the client through careful questioning. This process of guided discovery leads clients to greater clarity and understanding of their particular life situation.

Cognitive distortion is therefore often a target of intervention and may include the following:

- "I cannot be happy unless I have a child."
- "I am not as worthwhile as others who have children."
- "I am being punished."
- "I am not a real woman or man."

- "My body is betraying me."
- "My partner will not want me."

Candido and Candido emphasize that "it is important for the person to realize these thoughts are interpretations of their situation and not feelings. The feelings of depression, anxiety, and anger are influenced by the thoughts. People tend to confuse the two. Feelings are not facts." However, the therapist does not

> dismiss someone's very real and genuine feelings of sadness, regret, fear, and anger. The question is rather one of accuracy. Are they really useless because they cannot bear a child? Are they really incompetent because they cannot completely control their reproductivity? Are they really incapable of handling this situation? Really? Is bearing a child the most important element in their life or is the fulfillment of a core value in their life, such as the expression of love and the giving of oneself, the most important element? This is a chance for the individual to reexamine, reaffirm, and eventually celebrate their central values. This is an opportunity to find new ways of expressing those values and giving new life to what is truly important to them. Truly.

When employing cognitive therapy,

> sessions are structured and goal-oriented with the patient and therapist setting a collaborative agenda. Sessions begin with "What would you like to accomplish today?" Homework is then reviewed. There is a strong emphasis on in-between-session work. Infertile persons and couples may have various assignments ranging from the educational (for example, reading about aspects of infertility) to the therapeutic (for example, asserting oneself with physicians). The body of the agenda is then discussed with full utilization of cognitive therapy techniques, followed by a summarization and assignment of homework. Technique selection always derives from a collaborative conceptualization of the person(s) and their goals.

For most infertility patients like your client, cognitive therapy can be quite helpful and should offer some relief from their depression and anxiety. However, we caution you to temper your expectations of how much relief is possible with the knowledge that these symptoms are a normal part of the process of infertility. As such they often will ebb and flow based on the time of the woman's cycle (moods up at the beginning of the cycle when there is hope, and very low at the end with her period). Also affecting her moods will be her experiences with the outside world (such as pregnant women, advertisements for baby products, and family gatherings) and milestones such as holidays, birthdays, and anniversaries of losses.

Therefore we would not necessarily recommend medication unless

1. your client specifically requests it;
2. you feel the depression or anxiety becomes debilitating, preventing her from going to work; or doing other activities not involving pregnancy or small children;★ and/or
3. the depression becomes so serious that suicide becomes an issue.

If one or more of these factors are present, antidepressant medication can be used cautiously. We recommend that clients speak directly with their reproductive endocrinologist to discuss the effects of drug therapy on the infertility treatment and potential pregnancy. Or, if requested to do so, you should make your client's needs known to her physician.

No matter what method(s) you ultimately employ, help your client to see "that true hope is based on the belief that we do not know what the future holds. False optimism is based on a false belief that everything will be all right. Whether they will ever conceive or won't ever conceive is something that is simply not known and it is this inability to know the future upon which true hope rests."

5. How Can I Get My Client to Try Stress Reduction Techniques?

I have started seeing a woman who is in her mid-thirties and is currently undergoing treatment for infertility. Although she has been trying to get pregnant for the past three years, she has only recently sought out a specialist for medical treatment. In the course of our discussions, I have noticed very high levels of stress, which seems appropriate considering the pressure she is under. However, when I began to discuss this stress with her and suggested we explore some stress reduction techniques, she became very angry and has yet to answer any of my questions regard-

---

★ Many infertile women stop shopping in malls, food stores, and other public places perceived as minefields of pregnant women and baby strollers. Some women also choose to quit or take a leave of absence from their jobs as the pressures and demands of treatment increase. For infertile clients, some degree of avoidance, employment changes, and withdrawal can be expected and do not necessarily indicate that drug therapy is needed.

ing the reason for her strong response. I feel she needs help with her stress; however, I am reluctant to push this issue any further. Can you offer some insight into her reaction and suggest where I can go from here?

"Have a more positive attitude, quit your job, go on vacation, have a glass of wine. Relax, *relax*, RELAX . . ." If your client is like most infertility patients, she has probably been hearing these well-meaning suggestions for years from her family, friends, and possibly even her gynecologist. Unfortunately, however, these types of comments fall far short of good advice and often cause patients to feel guilty for not being able to relax *enough* to get pregnant. This may explain why your client responded so negatively to your suggestion that she try stress reduction techniques. She may have thought, albeit incorrectly, that you were like the others, that you believed if she were a more well-adjusted and relaxed person, she would not be infertile.

Your client's reaction, although understandable, has cut her off from further discussion and from the benefits of techniques that are invaluable for reducing the incredible stress infertility places upon women. Before considering how you can persuade your client to try stress reduction techniques, it is important to understand the nature of stress.

There has been much documentation of the relationship between stress and infertility in the last ten years.

> In a 1992 study of 338 infertile women and 39 matched fertile controls, the prevalence and predictability of depression were assessed. The infertile women had significantly higher depression scores than the control subjects and also had twice the prevalence of depressive symptoms. Infertile women are not only significantly more depressed than their fertile counterparts, their depression and anxiety levels are equivalent to women with heart disease, cancer or HIV-positive status.

Alice Domar, Ph.D., who has done extensive research in the field, believes the relationship between stress and infertility is a chicken-and-egg kind of situation; stress could be the cause of some infertility problems, and infertility problems, no matter what the origin, cause stress. If we know for certain that infertility puts enormous amounts of stress on the individual and couple, it makes sense to find ways to alleviate it.[21]

For example, some infertile patients enrolled in intensive stress management regimens like Domar's ten-week course at the Behavioral Medicine for Infertility program at New England Deaconess Hospital in Boston have shown startling results. "Of the 110 subjects who participated in the program and learned numerous relaxation techniques, 34 percent conceived within six months of completing the workshop. Of those who underwent an IVF cycle during or immediately following the completion of the program 37 percent conceived, twice the national rate."[22]

We believe Domar's findings are just the tip of the iceberg. The National Institutes of Mental Health are conducting a five-year study to establish whether it is possible to prevent depression in infertile women.[23] The American Society for Reproductive Medicine (ASRM) is also interested in learning more about the relationship between stress and fertility and has published many papers referring to the link.

Sybil Lefferts, C.S.W., a psychotherapist specializing in the mind/body connection, feels that those who learn basic relaxation techniques, the use of mental imagery, and other stress management strategies are better able to do the work of healing. She says the mind/body paradigm acknowledges that stress and illness are inseparable, an idea intrinsic to Eastern philosophies and healing methods, and only recently acknowledged in Western medicine.[24]

Today therapists and hospital and clinic programs that have incorporated stress management skills into their work have found them essential in helping their infertile patients manage their high anxiety. Peggy Bruhn, C.S.W., a psychotherapist specializing in loss and grief work, writes:

> I help my clients develop a "tool box." The box contains the ability to recognize messages sent from the body to the brain that signify stress, the skills necessary to breathe deeply and fully (many sessions are spent on teaching the clients to breathe in order to lessen anxiety), and the ability to talk to themselves about what they need, in the moment, to lessen their feelings of being out of control. The development of the contents takes patience, practice, and fine-tuning before the clients use it outside of the therapeutic milieu. They take their box with them to treatments, to baby showers, to the mall—really anywhere that is potentially stressful. I also ask my clients to imagine their favorite places and to "go there" during stressful times. As you can imagine, clients come up with their own ingenious, creative, and effective tools.

Bruhn also gives highly anxious clients a stone to keep with them as they journey through their infertility. The stone is always kept a "stone's throw" away, as a reminder that they have the "tools" they need to manage their anxiety in a health-sustaining way.[25]

It is important for therapists and other professionals working with infertile patients to familiarize themselves with healing techniques such as healthful breathing and meditation. But in order to teach a technique, one must know how to *do it*.[26] In Appendix I, we have provided various exercises to help you and your client learn these techniques. We also encourage you to read the work of Domar, Herbert Benson, and Jon Kabot-Zinn, Ph.D. Other well-known practitioners such as Joan Borysenko, Ph.D., and Belleruth Naparstek have published books, produced audiotapes, and appear regularly at conferences for both professionals and the general public.★

Once you feel comfortable with these techniques you can introduce stress management as part of your client's therapy by letting her know that you are not placing the blame for her infertility on her. Rather, you are trying to help her understand and get through what is considered to be one of life's worst crises.

6. How Will Narrative Therapy Help My Client Work Through an Adoption Loss?

A client I recently began seeing came into treatment because she was depressed. After years of infertility she and her husband decided to end medical treatment and pursue adoption. After three months of advertising they had what her lawyer considered to be a perfect situation: a young woman in her first year of college with no family support and a boyfriend who disappeared as soon as he found out she was pregnant. She expressed a strong desire to finish her education and believed adoption to be a positive solution. During the last six weeks of the pregnancy, my client had weekly phone visits and developed a good trusting rapport with the birth mother. She even went to the hospital and witnessed the birth of the baby.

But when my client arrived at the hospital the next day, the nurse on duty told her she and her husband would not be allowed to visit the baby. Her lawyer informed her that the birth mother's parents had had a change of heart after seeing the baby and had decided to lend support to their daughter. The adoption was off, and this couple was devastated.

That was two months ago. Since then my client has not gone back to work or

---

★ Alice Domar's studies can be found in the American Society for Reproductive Medicine's monthly journals from 1990 on. (See Appendix II for the address and phone number of the ASRM.) The References and Suggested Readings for Part V list printed works by Benson, Kabot-Zinn, Borysenko, and Naparstek.

resumed other more normal activities. She says she doesn't understand her lack of motivation and neither does anyone around her. Although her friends and family were supportive of her when she returned home empty-handed, they are now questioning why it's taking her so long to recover. I would like to help her get closer to what is really going on and am interested in knowing what approach you would use.

Adoption loss is a term we have coined to describe the experience of your client and the thousands of others who have suffered this type of devastating loss. Misunderstood in our society by most everyone including professionals, adoption loss leaves clients feeling "crazy" as they experience grief over a baby they have often never seen, held, or cared for.

To help couples feel entitled to their grief and to help them through this difficult time, therapists can employ the technique of *narrative therapy.* Narrative therapists such as Harry Rieckelman, L.C.S.W., M.F.A., Father Paul Costello, B.A., M.Ed., and Kathie Hepler, M.A., from the Institute for Narrative Therapy in Washington, D.C., look at the "stories" clients bring to them as constructs of their reality. These are not to be judged as fact or fiction by the therapist, but rather to be viewed as the clients' personal perception of the truth.[27]

Narrative therapy represents a new and innovative approach to treatment:

> It borrows from the constructivists in the field of literary criticism, where narratives are taken apart and analyzed for meaning, and from the social constructionists in the field of social psychology, where reality is viewed as coconstructed in the minds of individuals in interaction with other people and societal beliefs."[28]

Michael White and David Epston, the cofounders of the narrative therapy movement, believe that

> we all "story" our lives to make sense out of them. We cannot remember all of our lived experiences; there is too much material and too many many experiences unrelated to each other to retain it all, so our narrative structuring experience is a selective process. We arrange our lives into sequences and into dominant story lines to develop a sense of coherence and to ascribe meaning to our lives.[29]

In addition, the narrative approach works because, as Bill O'Hanolan writes in *Family Therapy Networker,* it leads to a vastly altered view of personality itself and therefore of therapeutic change. Many of the beliefs we cling to most dearly are nothing but a vast cultural rag bag: lines from old love songs, Glamour magazine layouts, movies, stern lectures from our fathers about what it is like to be a man [or woman]. We may have unconsciously absorbed beliefs that we aren't good enough, that worthwhile people know how to dress, only thin women are beautiful or worthy . . .[30]

and nonbiological parents have no right to feel love for a baby they did not bear.

These social constructs are what we internalize as the truth; they shape our identities and make our stories. For instance, one woman who suffered an adoption loss told the team of narrative therapists from Washington a story that began with hope.[31] She wanted to believe that the child she was going to adopt would be hers. She prepared for the baby's arrival, quit her job, decorated a nursery, shopped for baby clothes—in essence had an *adoption pregnancy*. She believed this adoption situation would not only end the infertility nightmare she was experiencing but would also change her and allow others to see her differently. Becoming a mother would redefine her; she would finally be like all the others around her—normal, functioning, and happy.

Yet everyone told her she should not bond with this unborn child, that she had no right to such strong emotions. They told her she should keep her feelings in check; after all, she had no biological ties to the child, and the situation was out of her control. The view that others held of her supported and validated parts of this woman's "old story" and the way she had defined herself before her experience with infertility. These old stories included themes underscored by failure, being different from others in her social network, and most of all being overreactive in situations (other than infertility) that seemed to others to be insignificant.

Sadly, the adoption story took a turn for the worse, when the birth mother told the client that she would not be this child's mother. Now she felt that all those people warning her had been right, that she must have been crazy for wanting this situation so badly. When all hope was dashed, the old story, with its theme of failure and unworthiness, rose again.

The narrative therapists' job was to break this pattern of internalizing negative events by externalizing the problem. So when the woman talked about the day she learned of her loss, the therapists needed to listen closely for the words she had chosen to "write" her adoption story with. They needed to find "the tiny hidden spark of resistance in her heart that was trapped in a label or diagnosis such as [overreactive or hysterical]"[32]—labels she had been given by others in her life, and which she had believed to be true.

My husband had just called the hospital to see when we could get our daughter and was told by the hospital social worker that the birth mother had taken the baby home. It was all over. I remember sitting there unable to move. I wanted to die. And then something came over me and I screamed. I screamed so loud that my goddaughter who lived across the street heard me and came running over. I couldn't walk, I couldn't do anything but scream the words, *"No! No!"* For the next two weeks I sat on the couch depressed, feeling as close to suicide as I have ever felt. I think I always knew from a place deep inside that it wouldn't work out. Not many things in my life work out. It was near Christmas and I could have cared less. I wanted to disappear. I wanted it all to go away.

After acknowledging that her story was devastating, the therapists wanted to talk more about this woman's response. The therapists questioned whether the phrase "screamed so loud that my goddaughter from across the street heard me" might have a different meaning than what the client believed. Instead of seeing her response as "overdramatic," they wondered if the loss of this baby had been so profound that, at the moment she heard the news, she had let out the primal scream of a mother who had lost her firstborn child. To this suggestion she replied, "Oh my God. I became a mother then, didn't I? The birth mother gave birth to me being a mother. That baby was mine, I loved her with all my heart, and now the birth mother has her. I would have been such a good mother to her. I pray to God the birth mother will do the same."

As this client became more and more comfortable with the new identity of mother, she was able to grieve the loss of her child. Regardless of what others said, she was now able to validate herself and her feelings and legitimize her sorrow. The therapists continued to work in collaboration with her to analyze the content and organization of her stories. As time went on, they began to challenge her negative self-concept. They could see the special significance she had given to certain life events that reinforced the images she held of herself.

As she was able to remember more lost fragments of experiences that proved her to be a survivor, a driven woman in the midst of authoring a new story, one of hope raised, hope dashed, and hope regained. Eventually she came to believe that she had a right to call herself a mother who had lost her first baby but desperately wanted another one. And so about six months later she and her husband went on to adopt a beautiful, healthy baby girl.

If you would like to know more about narrative therapy, the following articles and books are good resources:

- *The Family Therapy Networker,* vol. 18, no. 6 (November/December 1994), which has many excellent articles on narrative therapy
- Alan Parry and Robert E. Doan, *Story Revisions: Narrative Therapy in the Postmodern World* (The Guilford Press, New York, 1994)
- Hubert Hermans and Els Hermans-Jansen, *Self Narratives: The Construction of Meaning in Psychotherapy* (The Guilford Press, New York, 1995)
- Michael White and David Epston, *Narrative Means to Therapeutic Ends* (W. W. Norton & Company, New York, 1990)

7. Do Alternative Therapies Work with Infertility Clients?

I have been running an ongoing women's support group at a women's center for about two years. One member has been experiencing infertility since the group started. She got pregnant through artificial insemination but had a miscarriage toward the end of her first trimester.

She seems to be coping well, which could in part be due to the support she has sought out and received from the other group members. In fact, one woman who had experienced infertility told the group that she believed her problem conceiving stemmed from an unresolved conflict from a past life. Since she was able to get pregnant and have a child after her regression therapy, the other women in the group encouraged the infertile woman to seek out the same past-life therapist. Is there a place for this kind of treatment modality or for other alternative therapies when working with infertility clients? If so, what has been your experience with them?

Since conception is in reality a mystery beyond human control, the answer to the question "What helps?" cannot be solely grounded in the science of reproductive medicine. The proof of this lies in the simple truth that even today's medical specialists employing the best that science has to offer cannot predict which patient's cycle, or even which procedure, will be successful. As a society, we have allowed ourselves to believe that science has all the answers, even though statistics, especially those dealing with reproductive medicine, have proven this wrong.

While we would not encourage clients to abandon medical science, there is a growing body of evidence to suggest that, for some couples, alternative healing practices can be as successful as traditional medicine. At the very least, they are a valuable adjunct to current medical procedures. Much of the evidence for this is still anecdotal, as research in alternative approaches has attracted even less funding than traditional kinds of medical intervention. But as the safety of using drugs comes into question, as the costs of the high-tech treatments climb out of reach, and as insurance companies continue to limit coverage of reproductive services, patients continue to look for alternatives. Ironically, many of these alternatives come as gifts from our past. Stress management based on age-old traditions of meditation and visualization, as well as ancient healing practices such as acupuncture and herbal remedies, have all come into focus.

Thus it is not surprising that two of your clients have shown an interest in alternative therapies. For therapists working with infertility patients, practical knowledge of these alternatives is as important as understanding Western medical methods. However, it is not necessary for the therapist to be able to work in all treatment modalities. Referrals out to practitioners who specialize in alternative therapies are quite common; in most cases the relationship with the primary therapist can continue or pick up after adjunct treatments are completed. (Appendix II includes information on using naturopathic medicine and acupuncture for the treatment of infertility.)

To help clients uncover layers of unconscious thought patterns that may serve as roadblocks to both mental well-being and physical health, many therapists go beyond traditional talk therapy to include stress management, dream work, spiritual awareness, creative expression, bodywork, and past-life regression in their practices. Two such therapists who have helped infertility patients ease the burden of their treatments, heal their losses, and in some cases enhance their chances for a successful pregnancy, shared with us their thoughts.

Dr. Alla Renée Bozarth, director of Wisdom House in Oregon, is a soulcare giver, trained in Gestalt therapy and depth psychology. Here she describes her process with clients, which always begins with listening:

> I listen, as always, to the sacred story of the person who has come with this grief and longing, and I receive it with reverence. After that, a variety of approaches may follow—usually guided imagery that spirals down through layers of the psyche to the deepest roots of longing for a child. Often, this reveals an emotionally thwarted childhood on the part of the one who is longing, and we explore together the soul's longing for abundant welcome which was never given. It becomes understood that the person cannot freely and with integrity receive a child without first attending to the lost inner child—reaching out to her and welcoming her over time in many ways, including her in one's daily life, and

inviting her to come alive in one's soul with safety and acceptance promised. I serve as companion and guide in this process, teaching affirmations and offering practical suggestions for embracing the inner infant, toddler, child, and adolescent.[33]

During the course of her work with clients, Bozarth pays close attention to their dreams. Clients are asked to record their dreams in a journal which is then brought regularly to sessions for review:

We do intensive active imagination around sleep dreams and explore their meaning archetypally, as well as being receptive together for the gift of the Divine child which so often presents itself in dreams.

. . . I [also] encourage my clients to use various forms of creative expression throughout this process: I witness and receive and sometimes accompany the form, whether it is dance, song, painting, sculpting, poetry, weaving, or another form.

For those clients hoping to increase their chances for conception, the use of imagery may serve as an alternative or complement to medical treatment. Bozarth believes that imagery helps

the body open itself to conception. This also brings up unresolved childhood issues which are then addressed as I have described, while inviting the body to present spontaneous images of its own needs and desires. This becomes an important opportunity to explore the work of embodiment, to befriend the body and conceive of it in new, loving, and accepting terms. Tenderness and respect begin to replace negative body images or a refusal to live in the body, often resulting from childhood trauma, birth trauma, or some spiritual issue. These, then, become areas of exploration. Always, the soul is invited to tell its story through the body and imagination. I steadily extend this invitation.

Another area of exploration rarely talked about in relation to its effect on fertility is the experiences of past lives. For clients who are comfortable with the idea of reincarnation, past-life therapy can offer information that may lessen the anxiety felt in one's present life.

Roger J. Woolger, Ph.D., explains his view of past-life regression in his book *Other Lives, Other Selves: A Jungian Psychotherapist Discovers Past Lives*:

What past life remembering entails is a kind of deep identification with an inner or secondary personality, an identification which does indeed involve imagination, as all remembering does, but in the fullest sense. . . .

When we read novels or watch films and plays we practice varying degrees of this imaginative identification with the major characters; we are moved to terror or pity by imagining the story *as if* we were in their shoes, *as if* we were ourselves suffering their joys and sorrows. This is possible, psychologically, because we already have within us our own versions of these characters and their stories. . . . What past life remembering seems to do is bring these characters to the surface of consciousness with remarkable clarity, detail, and consistency by using the device of offering the psyche a blank screen called a "past life" to project them onto.[34]

Woolger emphasizes that *"it doesn't matter whether you believe in reincarnation or not* for past life therapy to be effective." Rather, he encourages his clients to believe in *". . . the healing power of the unconscious mind."*[35]

Sybil Lefferts, an educator and therapist trained in Ericksonian and Gestalt therapies, has worked with infertile women, including one who specifically expressed interest in using trancework as a path to her past-life experiences. Following is a brief summary of that therapeutic experience.

The client in question, an extremely spiritual woman, came to therapy with the belief that the soul chooses lifetimes in tune with what it needs to learn. From previous work done in past-life regressions, she had come to believe that her soul had always chosen bodies that were not fully functional.

After an initial in-take session of one hour, client and therapist met for seven two-hour sessions over a four-month period. During that time, the client always came prepared to work on a specific issue and thoughtfully continued to process the work between visits.

In the first regression, she was an unmarried woman who didn't want to become pregnant for fear of losing her attractiveness, becoming a burden, and being discarded by her lover. During the regression, the client reported being profoundly in touch with a fear of abandonment. She realized that although she truly wanted a child, some part of her did not. It was the first time she had understood this conflict.

In another regression she was a young woman in the court of a queen among dear women friends who had made a pact to remain single. She was forcefully taken away from her happy life by a suitor, whom she spurned. He then put her in a painful iron mask and she died young and childless. While reflecting on this session, the client felt that being childless and dying young in previous lives had yielded an important insight: a dimension of her current problem was not wanting to truly be a responsible adult. She also reported that the headache she had come in with that day was gone. (Interestingly, on later visits and following the end of treatment, the frequent headaches she had long suffered, had ceased.)

In succeeding regressions, she returned to lives in which she did have children. One of the most dramatic involved a lifetime in Nazi Germany, where she witnessed the murder of her child. This experience provided her with the insight that having a child in her current life would bring with it the fear of having to face such a loss. She had never considered this on a conscious level, and was impressed that it could have been such an important part of her unconscious makeup.

In her last session the theme of attachment versus independence reappeared. In her story, she was an independent, single man who prospered and lived to a ripe old age. Only on his peaceful deathbed, did he fleetingly feel remorse at being alone. In this trance state the client heard a woman's voice telling her that she had chosen that life to prove that she *could* be a loner. In future lives, although she would not be alone, a part of her would always remember this man and derive strength from him. In relating this to her real life, she spoke of the conflict between freedom and being unencumbered in younger years versus being alone and without children in old age.

The process of uncovering these "soul dramas" gave rise to complex feelings and led the client to confront many issues in her life. She realized that what she wanted was stirred into conflict with the needs of others, that she might not want to become a responsible adult, and that loving someone as much as she would love her child brings with it a fear of loss. Yet she also came to believe that life happens as it should, that all children have a time to be born, and that she must let go and be patient since the decision is really the child's. She realized that these beliefs sprang from a well of spirituality within her. She started to see life as a rushing stream, with humanity on a small raft which we have control over but which is riding a current moving in its own direction.

The client had a child about eight months after the last session. She believes the regression work was instrumental in helping her conceive, hold, carry, and deliver her healthy, wonderful baby.[36]

As more therapists and clients delve into this new form of treatment, past-life regression grows in both acceptance and popularity. This phenomenon has everything to do with both the changing belief systems of our culture as a whole and the positive effects this treatment has had on many of those willing to experience it.★

8. Does a History of Sexual Abuse Impact a Client's Reaction to Infertility?

I am seeing a woman who has three young children. She went through years of infertility to create her family: miscarriages, infertility treatments, and one life-threatening ectopic pregnancy. When she and her husband decided to adopt, she felt her dreams had finally come true. She loves staying home with her children and continues to be an excellent, devoted mother. In addition, she has a loving and supportive relationship with her husband, has good friends, and is thinking of returning to school to get a graduate degree in business. As she says, she couldn't ask for a better life.

Originally this woman came into treatment when her children were babies because she was experiencing episodes of anxiety for which she could find no explanation. As she began opening up, repressed memories of earlier sexual abuse began to surface, and we learned that there was a lot more to her story than we realized.

For years our treatment centered around issues relating to her early sexual abuse, but lately she is bringing up her infertility more and more. We have spent many sessions talking about her continued desire to experience a pregnancy even though she clearly does not want another baby and is very much in love with her three children. She cannot comfortably sit in a play group with pregnant women because, as she says, she feels different from them and wants to run out of the room whenever they talk about labor and delivery. She tells me she hardly ever feels like a "real woman." She also describes an overwhelming emptiness inside that nothing can fill—not her husband or her kids.

Are these symptoms common for women who have suffered from infertility? My gut tells me her reaction is extreme, but since I have not worked with many infertility patients, I am not sure.

Although infertility patients never lose the feelings associated with being infertile, over time these feelings lessen in intensity and move into the background of their lives. However, a number of issues, if not addressed, can cause women to keep infertility in the forefront and lead them to exhibit some of the more extreme symptoms your client is now reporting. Some of these issues, such as unresolved grief,

---

★ For further reading, we suggest Brian L. Weiss, M.D., *Many Lives, Many Masters* (Fireside, New York, 1988).

are discussed in this chapter; the Epilogue also goes into some detail about identity and the legacy of infertility.

One issue often overlooked regarding its impact on the infertility patient is sexual abuse in the client's background. While not all clients with this history will be affected, some—even those with repressed memories—are impacted more profoundly than the scarcity of literature on this issue might lead one to believe.

Through our discussions with sexually abused women, both fertile and infertile, we came to realize the impact childhood trauma can have on feelings about reproduction. For some who suffered abuse as a child, pregnancy can seem almost repulsive; the focus on their reproductive organs is a constant reminder of their traumatic history.

For other women, the experience of pregnancy can be life-affirming. The ability to relate to other women around pregnancy, childbirth, and breast feeding often has a significant and positive impact on their identities. In addition, self-esteem, a sense of purpose, and a positive body image may emerge during pregnancy. While not providing a complete healing, this is often their first opportunity to feel life where once there was only deadness. Some women even find themselves producing more children than they actually desire in an unconscious effort to continue re-creating this positive healing experience.

These benefits do not mean, however, that the total experience, especially the interactions with the medical community, is all positive. As we know, "The women who is on the doctor's examining table, feet in the stirrups, about to experience physical pain in the genital region at the hands of the physician, who is standing above her, is in a situation filled with the signs and signals of dominance, submission and a subtle message of threat."[37] For women who seek medical treatment for infertility, such images are repeated in their physician's office almost weekly, sometimes for years. Clearly such treatments have the potential of adding another layer of wounding to the psyches of abused women.

In addition to enduring the added intensity of medical treatment, the woman who remains infertile is deprived of the healing properties of a pregnancy. Feelings of being out of control, less of a woman, and different from everyone around her become personified. In some cases these feelings precipitate an unconscious, unceasing desire toward pregnancy as a way of healing. This desire may be so strong that the woman is unable to give up on the possibility of getting pregnant—even after exhausting all her emotional and financial resources and even after becoming a parent. Such may be the driving force behind your client's inability to let go of her fertile identity.

One woman said,

I wanted to be pregnant so bad, to experience life inside me and to breast-feed my baby. It's all I thought about. To be honest, I didn't know if I could do it—the breast feeding, I mean. I had a lot of trouble being touched there. It always felt uncomfortable. But I remember thinking that if I could breast-feed, maybe those feelings would go away forever and I would be cured. I don't know where this idea came from, and I never really thought about why I felt so uncomfortable in the first place.

It was not until after memories of early sexual abuse emerged that she understood where her intense yearnings and desires came from. Although she had not known that these "uncomfortable" sensations were rooted in past abuse, she nevertheless searched for a way to normalize these bodily feelings. This led her to pursue pregnancy at any cost. Had she not been infertile, the act of pregnancy and subsequent breast-feeding might have, to some extent, aided in her healing.

It is this yearning, this push of the psyche to look for health, that Gestalt therapist Joyce Magid talks about:

> The basic impulse of the human is our relentless moving forward toward the survival of our life force. Gestalt therapists believe in the intrinsic wisdom of the organism and the need and ability to experience our life force (sadness, joy, anger, love). Any interruption of a free flowing life force (which is our inherent birthright) and our interaction with our world, creates a diminished experience of life itself and can result in depression, anxiety, fear and unhappiness.
>
> . . . Gestaltists, working in the here and now of the therapy session, help the client experience fully her/his experiences. Beliefs are uncovered and challenged. Unshed tears of disappointment, unexpressed rage, buried terror, unaccessed love and softness—the stuff of life itself—emerge in the safe setting of a supportive therapeutic relationship.[38]

Within this relationship one can look for answers as to why a woman like your client would seem to be living two lives, one happy and gratified, the other unfulfilled and desirous of healing. In your mutual search for the missing pieces, remember that infertility by itself is never the whole story. Clients bring their entire history to bear on their infertility, not just their reproductive years. This history, both conscious and unconscious, can and does affect how the client approaches, feels about, and resolves her infertility. Only through this awareness, taking in the whole story, can the therapist help the client resolve those issues that continue to burden her long after she experiences the joys and fulfillment of parenthood.

PROFESSIONAL CONTRIBUTORS

ALLA RENÉE BOZARTH, Ph.D., is director of Wisdom House and one of the first women priests in the Episcopal Church, ordained in 1974. She is a widely published poet and soulcare giver. Trained in Gestalt Therapy and Depth Psychology she ministers to souls at Wisdom House in Western Oregon. Among her sixteen books and five audiotapes are *A Journey through Grief, Lifelines: Threads of Grace through Seasons of Change*, and *Love's Prism: Reflections from the Heart of A Woman,* including a chapter, "Letter to My Unborn Children."

PEGGY BRUHN, R.N., C.S.W., is a clinical social worker specializing in loss and bereavement. She was cofounder of Healthhouse, a women's health and resource center on Long Island. Bruhn also cofounded Reach-out to the Parents of an Unknown Child, a community-based support group for parents who have experienced miscarriage, stillbirth, or neonatal death. Bruhn has authored numerous articles on various forms of loss and bereavement and lectures locally and nationally on topics related to loss.

DOMINIC CANDIDO, Ph.D., is director of the Long Island Center for Cognitive Therapy, Oyster Bay and West Islip, New York, and is a clinical instructor in Psychiatry and Behavioral Sciences School of Medicine, University at Stony Brook, Stony Brook, New York. He is also a past Fellow at the Center for Cognitive Therapy at the University of Pennsylvania.

TERESA CANDIDO, C.S.W., A.C.S.W., is assistant director for the Long Island Center for Cognitive Therapy, Oyster Bay and West Islip, New York.

FATHER PAUL COSTELLO, B.A., M.Ed., B.Div., is an Australian Catholic priest, teacher, and writer specializing in narrative theory and literary practice. He is cofounder of the Institute for Narrative Therapy.

Having recently completed his graduate studies, he is now working as codirector of a think tank organization in Washington called The Narrative Institute where he continues to translate the breakthroughs of narrative method into broader areas of application, such as pastoral counseling, community renewal, mediation, organizational development, and spiritual guidance.

He is writing a book based on the narrative research of the institute and edits a journal, soon to be launched, called *Narrative Matters.*

DAVID ECKERT, Psy.D., is a clinical psychologist with a certificate in family therapy. Eckert works with children and families in both schools and private practice. He has led numerous workshops on issues relating to infertility and adoption.

Susan Gardner, C.S.W., B.C.D., is a support group leader for RESOLVE of Long Island in New York. She treats both primary and secondary infertility clients but specializes in working with secondary infertility clients.

Randi Guggenheimer, R.N., C.S.W., maintains a private psychotherapy and supervision practice in Syosset, New York. She is formally assistant director to Nassau County Services for Rape Victims. Guggenheimer has lectured extensively to the public on topics relating to women's issues.

Sonia Hieger, C.S.W., B.C.D., has a psychotherapy private practice and is a support group leader for RESOLVE of Long Island. She is also a trainer for volunteers and professionals as well as an advisor to the board of RESOLVE. Heiger is a member of the Long Island Institute for Psychoanalysis, the National Association of Social Workers, and the American Fertility Society.

Ira Kalina, Ph.D., is the director of Couple Works, a private marital therapy center on Long Island. He is past president of the Long Island chapter of the American Association of Marriage and Family Therapy (AAMFT) and is an Approved Supervisor of that national organization. Kalina has been training, supervising, and teaching couples therapy for over twenty years.

Sybil Lefferts, C.S.W., B.C.D., has a twenty-year interest in and experience with the body/mind connection. She was the project director and editor of three editions of the Suffolk County *People's Guide to Health Care.* She founded and supervised the Wellness Project, a publicly funded project providing counseling and wellness services to seniors and their families. She is in private practice in East Setauket, New York.

Joyce Magid, M.S.R., C.S.W., is a New York State–licensed psychiatric social worker. She is a psychotherapist and supervisor in private practice in New York City and Long Island working with individuals, couples, families, and groups for the past eighteen years. She is a leader of intensive residential therapy weekends, working primarily in the Gestalt modality. Magid is director of training for, and on the faculty and training staff of, the Gestalt Center of Long Island. A graduate of Queens College and Stony Brook University's School of Social Work, she also graduated from the Gestalt Center of Long Island Certificate Training Program and completed the Gestalt Institute of Cleveland's Intensive Couple and Family Training Program.

Nancy Newman, M.S.W., is a Family Therapist with a specialty in infertility. She has a private practice in British Columbia and Washington state, and teaches at a community college. She is authoring two books, *Commonly Asked Questions about IVF and Related Technologies* and *From the Heart: Stories of Open Adoption,* both to be published by University of Toronto Press in 1998.

HARRY RIECKELMAN, L.C.S.W., M.F.A., is a published story writer and director of the Institute for Narrative Therapy, Washington, D.C. He conducts one-day workshops and retreats on the theory and practice of narrative therapy. He has a private practice in Cabin John, Maryland.

LINDA SALZER, L.C.S.W., A.C.S.W., former president of the northern New Jersey chapter of RESOLVE, is currently in private practice in Englewood, New Jersey. She is the author of *Surviving Infertility* as well as numerous articles on infertility and adoption. Salzer contributes regularly to the *National RESOLVE Newsletter*'s "Ask the Expert" column. She speaks nationally to professional and consumer groups on the issues relating to infertility and adoption.

SHERYL STERN, M.A., received her master's degree in Creative Arts Therapy from Hofstra University and interned at North Shore University Hospital (Manhasset, N.Y.), Department of Psychiatry. She has conducted workshops for women with problems associated with infertility. In addition to being a telephone counselor for RESOLVE, she is coauthor of an article on the use of art therapy methodology with women facing fertility problems.

APPENDICES

APPENDIX I

SELF-HELP GUIDE

In this section, we describe the stress reduction techniques and exercises that have helped many infertility patients feel better physically and more in control emotionally. If you decide to try one of the methods, we suggest you begin slowly and practice without putting too much pressure on yourself. Seeing each exercise as an enjoyable and growthful experience will help you to incorporate them into your daily life. Remember that changing the way you deal with stress during this crisis can set the tone and pace for managing stress for the rest of your life.

BREATHING

For centuries, people who practiced yoga, T'ai Chi, prayer, meditation, and athletics understood that controlled and focused breathing reduced the negative effects stress had on their bodies. They learned that simple diaphragmatic breathing (as opposed to breathing from the chest) had the power to release anxiety and tension while it elicited more centered and clear thinking.

To understand how powerful the breath is and how closely your mind and body are linked, think about how your breathing changes when something excites, angers, or surprises you. Most of us take rapid, shallow breaths when angry. When surprised, we hold our breath and our heart races in excitement. When happy and content, our breathing is deep and full. We are usually not conscious of our bodies during these moments; we react automatically, not mindfully.

By becoming conscious of your breath, you can control this involuntary response and alter your reaction to stress (really *dis*tress). Imagine for a moment that you are in the middle of an argument with your spouse with all its anger and confusion. What do you think would happen if you became conscious of your breath, slowed it down—"took a breather" as they say. Your anxiety would most likely lessen, and you would be able to think, speak, and react more clearly.

Herbert Benson, M.D., and Eileen M. Stuart, R.N., M.S., in *The Wellness Book,* explain one way you can learn to breathe healthfully:

[Lie] on your back in a comfortable position. Close your eyes and place one hand on your belly just below the navel (belly button). Because of the movement of the diaphragm with each breath, as you inhale your hand will rise slightly. As you exhale, your hand will fall. Focus your attention on the rising and falling of your hand. This is diaphragmatic breathing. An ideal time to practice this is just before going to sleep. You can also practice it during the day when you are standing or sitting.

Another place to focus on breathing is at the nostrils. Observe how the air is slightly cooler as it enters your nose and somewhat warmer as it leaves.

Try a deep breathing exercise now. First sit comfortably in a chair or lie on the floor and close your eyes. Take several deep diaphragmatic breaths. As you continue to breath diaphragmatically, begin to count down on each outbreath, starting with ten and proceeding down to one. As you exhale, imagine the tension draining out of your body from head to toe. And allow your state of letting go to deepen gradually with each outbreath.[1]

VISUALIZATION OR GUIDED IMAGERY

These two terms, used interchangeably, refer to a technique many infertile people have found helpful for identifying and changing negative thoughts and feelings and for managing pain during difficult medical treatments. Aline P. Zoldbrod, Ph.D., in her pamphlet entitled, *Getting around the Boulder in the Road: Using Imagery to Cope with Fertility Problems,* explains that we all have the ability to think in words and concepts (or images). When you become conscious of your inner pictures, you can actually reprogram the disconcerting ones with positive and pacifying images. For instance, if you are nervous about a future doctor's appointment, you will note to yourself, "I have an appointment with the doctor at 2:00 tomorrow afternoon. I wonder what will happen? I wonder what she will tell me?" While you are silently saying these words, you might visualize yourself sitting anxiously in the waiting room, tapping your foot, running your fingers through your hair, or leafing through a magazine unable to concentrate on what you are reading. You feel so anxious that your stomach feels as if it is "tied up in knots." You don't consciously tell yourself to feel uncomfortable or to picture these scenes that cause anxiety; they just appear in your mind, unannounced.[2]

Zoldbrod suggests that visualization, like breathing, can work to transform these anxiety-ridden images to more calm and serene pictures. For example, by imagining you are untying the knot inside you and seeing your insides becoming unraveled and less anxious, you might be able to see yourself calmly waiting to see your physician. You imagine yourself reading a book that you enjoy, listening to peaceful music through head phones, or taking deep breaths with your hands on you abdomen as you bide your time.[3]

Another way to use visualization is to create new pleasurable images in your mind's eye. You can also call upon these comforting pictures when you have to get through an uncomfortable situation like a difficult medical procedure.

Belleruth Naparstek, author of *Staying Well with Guided Imagery,* describes a popular visualization entitled "Favorite Place Imagery." Our version of it, which follows, has been altered to fit the needs of infertility patients, who report using it successfully during IVF procedures and other difficult treatments.[4]

While you are practicing at home, make sure you will not be distracted: turn off your phone and television, and even put a "do not disturb" sign on your front door. Some patients play soft instrumental music in the background in order to enhance the visualization mood. We suggest, however, that you read through the exercise first to see whether you would like to use music or not. You may also want to record the words on a tape player so that you can play it for yourself whenever you wish.

Find a comfortable place to sit or lie down and adjust your body until you feel comfortable, trying not to cross your arms or legs. See if you can keep your head, neck, and body aligned. Place your hands gently on your stomach and when you are ready, close your eyes.

Take a full, deep breath (described above), inhaling as deeply as you can. Make sure that the breath does not stop in your chest. Push it down, all the way down to your abdomen. Feel your stomach rise and fall with each breath. Imagine a balloon filling with air on the inhale and deflating on the exhale. Slowly breath in and out, in and out, and feel your hands rise and fall with each breath.

Imagine that when you inhale you are sending your breath to all the tense places in your body. Imagine that the breath has a color soothing to you. And as you breathe, send the colored breath to all the places in your body that need comfort. Feel them loosen and soften as you allow your breath to fill each part. Push the breath all the way down to your toes. Allow the breath to fill each toe. Watch it in your mind's eye as it fills your ankles, calves, knees, thighs, pelvis, chest, shoulders, arms, back up into your neck, head, scalp, and face. Allow the breath to soften and loosen all the tenseness in your body. Imagine feeling safe and secure as the breath fills you. Remember to let the chair or bed support you, to let yourself go and feel the tension go from your body as you inhale and exhale.

When thoughts come to your mind, send them out with your breath. Watch them go. See them come in one side of your head and out the other. Let the thought float by your mind's eye each time you exhale. Feel your mind empty, even if only for a moment. Feel yourself being open and still.

Now, imagine you are getting into a vehicle of your choice. It can be a sports car, jeep, luxury car, motorcycle, bicycle—any vehicle that you want. When you get in or on it, let it take you to a place that you've always wanted to go. A place that feels safe and peaceful. It can be a real place, a fantasy place, anywhere that you want to go.

When you get to your safe place, get out of the vehicle and walk around. Look around, see what is there. Look in front of you, behind, up and down, to the right and the left. Listen to the sounds. Are there sounds in the background? Feel the air on you: is it warm, cold, wet, dry? What can you smell—the sweet scent of the air, the salt from the water? Is the sun out? Can you feel it on your body? Are you standing, sitting, or lying down? Fill each of your senses.

Let yourself be comforted in this place. Take a deep breath. Feel the breath as it goes down into your stomach. Feel your stomach rise and fall. Let the breath go all the way down to the tips of your toes and come all the way up to the top of your head. Feel the center of your body sink into the chair, bed, or floor. Let every muscle feel your breath as you take in all the beauty, all the peacefulness, of your safe place.

Let yourself be surrounded by your breath, your peaceful energy. Feel the quiet of your body and of your breath, in and out, in and out. Sit for a while more in this place and relax. You deserve it. You need to be here. You need the peacefulness of a quiet, safe place. Take it in. Feel your aliveness, your specialness, your strength. In and out, in and out, in and out . . .

When you are ready, you can open your eyes slowly. Take in all the you have experienced. Take in your ability to go to this safe place whenever you'd like.

MEDITATION

Meditation is another stress reduction technique that allows the body and mind to quiet down. Rather than creating an inner image to alter negative thoughts as in visualization, the meditator elicits the relaxation response by repeating a simple word or phrase or reflecting on an object. (That is not to say that a visualization or image will not occur during meditation; it is just not the overall goal.)

Alice Domar, Ph.D., director of the Infertility Program at the Mind/Body Medical Institute of New England Deaconess Hospital, has found meditation to be extremely helpful for patients experiencing the emotional and physical roller-coaster ride of infertility. After patients learn to breathe deeply and fully, and obtain a relaxed response, she encourages them to use meditation. Domar instructs her patients to focus on a comforting word or phrase. She suggests using a Sanskrit mantra of *Ham Sah* (*Ham* means "I am," and *Sah* means "that"). Other words like *Om,* or "peace/ful," can be used.[5]

As in the breathing and visualization exercises above, find a comfortable spot in a quiet place. You can either sit or lie down, close your eyes or keep them open—whatever makes you most comfortable.

> As you breathe in, begin to concentrate on the word Ham (pronounced "Haam") in your mind. Let the sound reverberate, like the Hmmm feeling you get when you sink into a hot bath. As you exhale, concentrate on the word Sah (pronounced "Saah") in your mind like a sigh. Do this for several moments. (Inhale through your nose and exhale through your mouth, if that is most comfortable.)
>
> If your attention wanders, gently bring it back to Ham as you inhale, and Sah as you exhale.[6]

Meditation, when practiced over a period of time, has given many infertility patients the calm and peace they need to get through stressful treatments. One patient who was claustrophobic told us she had put off having a necessary MRI because she believed she would have an anxiety attack during the procedure. After practicing meditation on a daily basis, she was able to make her way through the examination.

PHYSICAL EXERCISE

Most physicians feel exercise is an excellent way to decrease the anxiety and depression so often experienced in infertility. They encourage patients to *continue* their usual routines or if desired to begin gentle exercising such as walking, swimming, or bicycling. However, any *new* routine that requires intense strenuous exercise is discouraged.★

All patients taking fertility drugs have to be particularly sensitive to their bodies immediately after ovulation since there is a risk of ovarian rupture after stimulation. During this time, patients are encouraged to stop all exercise if they feel even the slightest twinge of pain or bloating.

JOURNAL KEEPING AND WRITING

The daily ritual of writing down thoughts and feelings is one way to discover, explore, and become privy to your innermost feelings. Many infertility patients experiencing confusing thoughts and feelings have found it helpful to journal.

★ Some avid athletes have found their menstrual cycles interrupted or completely stopped, especially when training for competition. If this occurs, it is vital that you let your physician know.

We encourage you to buy a special book and a special pen to write with, and to pick a separate place that makes you feel safe and far enough away from interruptions to write confidentially and truthfully. One patient we knew began by writing "I hate infertility" over and over again. That one repetitive thought spurred her to break through her anger to the feelings underneath. Through writing she discovered she was sad and frustrated and that she was unwilling to continue treatment with her physician. She got a second opinion and resumed treatment with another group of specialists whose treatment plans were more aligned with her philosophy.

Other infertility patients have used their journals to keep track of their menstrual cycles, drugs, treatments, and pregnancy test outcomes. We encourage you to record these events and to write down the feelings associated with each experience.

DAILY INFERTILITY LISTS

One way to feel more in control during a crisis is to become organized. Create a daily "things to do" list that includes phone calls, errands, or appointments. Next to each item, jot down when the best time would be to complete the task. Try to prioritize your time so that your infertility chores do not overlap and interfere with other aspects of your life. (See Chapter 5.)

FOCUSING

If you find your thoughts of infertility invading your mind so much that you are unable to concentrate, try a focusing exercise. Many people experiencing infertility have used this exercise to counteract chronic daydreaming as they drive, work, read, or watch television.

For example, if you feel yourself drifting while driving, take a deep breath and say to yourself, "I am driving in my car. My hands are on the steering wheel, my foot is on the gas pedal. I have the radio on and it is playing———. The windows are down. I can feel the wind on my arm, in my hair. I am wearing my jeans and a T-shirt, and I have my sneakers on. I was just thinking about my doctor's appointment, but now I must get back to driving and look at the road."

APPENDIX II

RESOURCE DIRECTORY

FOR GENERAL INFERTILITY
AND OTHER HEALTH-RELATED ISSUES

American Association of Marriage and Family Therapists
1133 15th Street N.W.
Suite 300
Washington, DC 20005-2710

(202) 452-0109; (800) 374-2638
Web site: *http://www.aamft.org*

Provides information and referrals to marriage and family counselors.

American College of Obstetricians and Gynecologists
409 12th Street S.W.
Washington, DC 20024-2188

(202) 638-5577

More than 33,000 physicians specializing in obstetric-gynecologic care are members. The college keeps members informed about care standards based on most recent scientific research.

American Society of Andrology
74 New Montgomery
Suite 230
San Francisco, CA 94105

(415) 764-4822
E-mail: *105037.1120@compuserve.com*

Provides referrals to urologists and andrologists in your area.

American Society for Reproductive Medicine (ASRM)
1209 Montgomery Highway
Birmingham, AL 35216-2809

(205) 978-5000
E-mail: *asrm@asrm.com*
Web site: *http://www.asrm.com*

Professional organization dedicated to advancing knowledge and expertise in reproductive medicine and biology. Will provide patients with referrals to members. Publications include a monthly medical journal, guidelines for practicing clinicians, ethics reports, and numerous patient information fact sheets and pamphlets. Topics cover adolescent gynecology, prevention of sexually transmitted diseases, infertility diagnosis and treatment, assisted reproductive technology, and menopause. Health policy, legislation, and media relations are handled by the Washington office. The organization's 10,000 members include ob/gyns, reproductive endocrinologists, nurses, urologists, andrologists, psychologists, social workers, research scientists, and other health-care professionals.

DES Action
1615 Broadway
#510
Oakland, CA 94612

(800) DES-9288
E-mail: *desaact@well.com*
Web site: *http://www.desactction.org*

Consumer group for people exposed to DES (diethylstilbeshol) during their mother's pregnancy. The organization publishes a quarterly newsletter and offers special publications including a fertility and pregnancy guide. A national referral physician list is available, as are legal referrals.

Endometriosis Association
8585 N. 76th Place
Milwaukee, WI 53233

(800) 992-3636

An international self-help nonprofit organization providing support and education for patients with endometriosis and their families, and performs research on the disease.

FERRE Institute
258 Genesee Street
Suite 302
Utica, NY 13502

(315) 724-4348

Provides infertility education programs, publishes brochures, sponsors conferences, and offers a lending library containing literature on infertility-related issues; will also loan books by mail.

Ovarian Cancer Registry
Gilda Radner Familial
Roswell Hurk Cancer Institute
Buffalo, NY 14263

800-OVARIAN

Provides information on the risk factors and diagnostic tests for ovarian cancer. The registry is for families with a history of ovarian and/or breast cancers. Provides referrals to physicians, support groups, and a help line for women who have had or are contemplating an oophorectomy.

Hysterectomy Educational Resources and Services (HERS)
422 Bryn Mawr Avenue
Bala Cynwd, PA 19004

(610) 667-7757

A nonprofit women's health organization providing information on the alternatives to hysterectomy, surgerical information, and referrals to physicians worldwide. HERS offers free counseling to women by telephone, by appointment.

Infertility and Pregnancy Loss (INCIID Links and Online Resources)
P.O. Box 3863
Arlington, VA 22206

(703) 379-9178; (520) 544-9548
Web site: *http://www.inciid.org*
email: *nancy@inciid.org*

A nonprofit, consumer-oriented organization that provides links to the latest information on the Internet about the many types of infertility that can impede a couple's ability to have children. Care has been taken to provide links to only those Web sites and articles that offer accurate, medically responsible points of view and reviewed by qualified physicians or therapists. Twenty-five facts sheets on specific subjects are available, as well as a directory of professionals according to geographic location. This cyberspace organization offers professionally moderated bulletin boards on specific subjects of interest to people experiencing infertility.

National Society of Genetic Counselors
233 Canterbury Drive Box I.B.
Wallingford, PA 19086

(610) 872-7608

Will send free brochure about genetic counselors who specialize in infertility. Brochures are also available in Spanish. The society does not maintain or disseminate information about specific genetic disorders.

National Women's Health Network
514 10th Street N.W.
Suite 400
Washington, D.C. 20004

(202) 347-1140

An organization seeking to give women a greater voice in the health-care system in the United States. It directs people and policies toward responsible, humane health care, educates women about health care to make them better-informed health-care consumers, and monitors health-related legislation to protect women's health rights. An information packet on infertility is available by calling or writing.

North American Menopause Society
P.O. Box 94527
Cleveland, Ohio 44101-4527

(216) 844-8748

Offers a suggested reading list and referrals to physicians and support groups. Has published ten books on menopause-related issues. Prefers to receive requests via mail.

RESOLVE
1310 Broadway
Somerville, MA 02144-1731

Help line: (617) 623-0744
E-mail: *resolveinc@aol.com*
Web site: *http://www.resolve.org*

A national organization, with local chapters in most states, whose mission is to provide timely, compassionate support and information to people experiencing infertility and to increase awareness of infertility issues through advocacy and public education. Membership includes subscription to a national newsletter, discounts on literature, and access to medical information including referrals to support groups and local chapters.

Serona Symposia, USA, Inc. (SSUSA)
100 Longwater Circle
Norwell, MA 02061

(800) 283-8088

An independent, nonprofit corporation funded by Serona Laboratories, Inc., SSUSA is dedicated to excellence in continuing health education and has a long-term commitment to physician, health-care, professional, and patient education. SSUSA cosponsors educational conferences.

Women's Health Connection
P.O. Box 6388
Madison, WI 53716-0338

(800) 366-6632

A consumer health education resource network dedicated to educating women about hormone-related disorders such as PMS, menopause, infertility, and postpartum depression. Publishes a newsletter that highlights articles on current women's health topics and hormone disorders.

ALTERNATIVE HEALTH CARE

American Association of Naturopathic Physicians

2366 East Lake Avenue
Suite 322
Seattle, WA 98102

(206) 324-7610

Will give referrals. Naturopathic physicians are not licensed to practice in all states; however, they practice in most parts of the United States.

American Association of Oriental Medicine (AAOM)

433 Front St.
Catasauqua, PA 18032

(610) 266-1433

The largest professional organization organized to further the development of oriental medicine as a complementary field of health care in America. For a referral to a qualified practitioner in your area, call AAOM. Referrals are to practitioners who are certified or licensed in their state.

Homeopathic Academy of Naturopathic Physicians (HANP)

P.O. Box 12488
Portland, OR 97212

(503) 795-0579

Provides free of charge a directory of naturopathic physicians board-certified in homeopathy.

National Center for Homeopathy (NCH)

801 North Fairfax Street
Suite 306
Alexandria, VA 22314

(703) 548-7790

E-mail: *nchinfor@igc.apc.org*
Web site: *http://www.homeopathic.org*

Dedicated to promoting homeopathy through education, information, publication, and membership services. Each spring the NCH holds a national conference on homeopathy, and every summer it conducts a training program with courses for professionals and consumers. Membership is $40.

National Certification Commission for Acupuncture and Oriental Medicine

P.O. Box 97075
Washington D.C. 20090-7075

(202) 232-1404

Provides list of certified acupuncturists and herbalists. Send check or money order for $3.00 for each state listing.

Spindrift Foundation

P.O. Box 5134
Salem, OR 97304-5134

An organization that conducts scientific experiments on the effects of prayer on healing.

ADOPTION

Adoption Assistance Services

Readers interested in initiating adoption benefits in their workplace can obtain valuable resources and direction from the three organizations listed below. Samples of corporate adoption policies, request letters for adoption assistance, and a listing of corporations that offer adoption assistance are just some of the services the following organizations offer.

Dave Thomas Foundation for Adoption

Box 7164
Dublin, OH 43017

(614) 764-8454

National Adoption Center—Adoption Benefits Coordinator

1500 Walnut Street
Suite 701
Philadelphia, PA 19102

(215) 735-9988

Adoptive Families of America (AFA)

2309 Como Avenue
St. Paul, MN 55108

(612) 645-9955
(800) 372-3300
Web site:*http://www.adoptive fam.org*

The largest nonprofit organization in the United States serving adoptive and prospective adoptive families. The AFA is a membership organization of 20,000 families and more than 200 adoptive parent support groups in the United States and around the world all committed to building families through adoption. The AFA seeks to create opportunities for successful permanent families for children through education, advocacy, and support. The organization publishes a national bimonthly magazine *Adoptive Families,* which contains current adoption news and parenting issues. The AFA has a help line (612-535-4829) to assist you with any questions.

American Academy of Adoption Attorneys

P.O. Box 33053
Washington, DC 20053-0053

(202) 832-2222

A national organization of attorneys who practice or have otherwise distinguished themselves in the field of adoption law. The academy's work includes promoting the reform of adoption law and disseminating information on ethical adoption practices. Publishes newsletter and educational open seminars. Send request to the academy for a directory of their members according to geographic area. .

Families for Private Adoption

P.O. Box 6375
Washington, DC, 20015-0375

(202) 722-0338

Supports and educates families who are interested in private, non-agency adoption. Helps families to network with other adoptive families as well as other adoption organizations. Conducts a fall and spring workshop entitled "Successful Private Adoptions" which covers issues on the legalities of adoption, the how-to's of advertising, and birth parent perspectives.

La Leche League

1400 N. Meachum Rd.
Schaumburg, IL 60168-4079

(800) LALECHE

Web site: *http://www.lalecheleague.org*

Will supply names of La Leche groups in your community. Biological and adoptive mothers interested in nursing can find information and support.

National Adoption Center

1500 Walnut Street
Suite 701
Philadelphia, PA 19102

(215) 735-9988

An organization devoted to helping children with special needs and from minority cultures to find loving homes. The center is not an agency; that is, they do not have children in their care. They do, however, work closely with agencies all over the country to offer information and referrals.

National Council on Adoption
1930 17th Street, N.W.
Washington, DC 20009

(202) 328-1200

Serves children needing families, adoptive families, and women facing the difficult decisions that accompany an unplanned pregnancy. Publishes reports on adoption issues such as open records, interracial adoption, and legislation affecting adoptees.

North American Council on Adoptable Children
970 Raymond Avenue
Suite 106
St. Paul, MN 55114-1149

(612) 644-3036

Conducts research, education, and outreach activities related to adoption, particularly of children with special needs; holds an annual conference; publishes a quarterly newsletter; engages in research; publishes findings about topics that relate to foster care and adoption; and supports the work of adoptive parents groups.

Perspectives Press
P.O. Box 90318
Indianapolis, IN 46290-0318

(317) 872-3055
Web site: *http://www.perspectivespress.com*

Publishes books on adoption and infertility-related issues for children and parents. A catalog is available.

CHILD-FREE LIVING

Childfree Network
6966 Sunrise Blvd.
Suite 111
Citrus Heights, CA 95610

(916) 773-7178

A national organization that provides education, support, and resources for child-free individuals and couples. For information and a sample newsletter, send a self-addressed stamped envelope with $0.55 return postage to address listed above.

PREGNANCY

Center for Multiple Births
333 East Superior Street
Room 464
Chicago, IL 60611

(312) 266-9093

Will send resources.

La Leche League
1400 N. Meachum Rd.
Schaumburg, IL 60168-4079

(800) LALECHE
Web site: *http://www.lalecheleague.org*

Will supply names of La Leche groups in your community. Biological and adoptive mothers interested in nursing can find information and support.

Mothers of Supertwins (MOST)
P.O. Box 951
Brentwood, NY 11717

(516) 434-MOST

A national support network for families who are expecting, or who are already the parents of, triplets or more. One of the primary goals of MOST is to help families make informed decisions regarding their pregnancy and their children's development. Counseling is also available for families considering aggressive fertility measures.

Sidelines

P.O. Box 1808
Laguna, CA 92652

(714) 497-2265

Provides support, education, and advocacy to women with high-risk pregnancies and their families, with Community-based chapters throughout the United States. It publishes *Left Sidelines* for women with complicated pregnancies and is very sensitive to the issues surrounding pregnancy following infertility.

The Twin to Twin Transfusion Syndrome Foundation

411 Longbeach Parkway
Bay Village, OH 44140

(216) 899-8887
Fax (216) 899-1184

Dedicated to providing educational, emotional, and financial support to families and caregivers before, during, and after pregnancies with Twin to Twin Transfusion Syndrome. Special support to families experiencing loss as well as families with children with physical challenges.

Organizations Dealing with Third-Party Reproduction

American Surrogacy Center

638 Church Street N.E.
Marietta, GA 30060

(770) 426-1107
Web site: *http://www.surrogacy.com*

Has a Web site for surrogacy and egg donation as well as infertility-related E-mail discussion groups. Membership is free, and no one is allowed in discussion groups unless they have had experience with the issues being discussed. Live twenty-four-hour chats and monthly virtual seminars with top professionals in the field.

Options—National Fertility Registry

11947 Valley View Street
#6209
Garden Grove, CA 92845

(310) 404-5035; (800) 786-1786

National database containing comprehensive profiles and photographs of egg donors, sperm donors, and surrogates throughout the United States.

Parenting

Mothers of Supertwins (MOST)

P.O. Box 951
Brentwood, NY 11717

(516) 434-MOST

A national support network for families who are expecting, or who are already the parents of multiples (triplets or more). One of the primary goals of MOST is to help families make informed decisions regarding their pregnancy and their children's development. Counseling is also available for families considering aggressive fertility measures.

National Organizations of Mothers of Twins Club, Inc.

P.O. Box 23188
Albuquerque, NM 87192-1188

(800) 243-2276

A support group of parents of twins and higher-order multiples. It provides referrals to local support groups and an informational brochure, *Your Twins and You.*

Loss Support Organizations .

CLIMB—Center for Loss in Multiple Births

P.O. Box 1064
Palmer, AK 39645

(907) 746-6123

Publishes quarterly newsletter and contact list for parents who have lost one or more babies. Samples of birth and memorial announcements available.

Compassionate Friends

P.O. Box 3696
Oak Brook, IL 60522–3996

(630) 990–0010

An international organization offering friendship and understanding to parents and siblings who have lost a child regardless of age or cause of death.

Pregnancy and Infant Loss Center

1421 E. Wayzata Blvd.
Suite 30
Wayzata, MN 53391

(612) 473–9372

A nonprofit organization providing support, resources, and education to families suffering from miscarriage and stillbirth.

Pregnancy Loss Support Program for Miscarriage, Stillbirth, and Newborn Death

9 East 69th Street
New York, NY 10021

(212) 535–5900

A nonsectarian project of the National Council of Jewish Women.

SHARE

St. Joseph Health Center
300 First Capitol Drive
St. Charles, MO 63301–2893

(314) 947–4747
Web site: *http://www.nationalshareoffice.com*

National organization that provides support, counseling, assistance, and resources for bereaved families who have lost infants and newborns due to miscarriage, stillbirth, or neonatal death. Publications are available.

Sudden Infant Death Syndrome (SIDS)

1314 Bedford Avenue
Suite 210
Baltimore, MD 21208

(800) 221–SIDS
E-mail: *sidshq@charm.net*

An organization that provides information on infant loss and makes referrals to a nationwide network of parent support programs. Publishes a free brochure. Also has a national toll-free hot line, staffed twenty-four hours with a counselor.

NOTES

1 Who Am I?

1. Ruthellen Josselson, *Finding Herself* (Jossey-Bass Publishers, San Francisco, 1987), p. 171.
2. Many of the ideas in the answer to this question are taken from Matthew McKay, Peter D. Rogers, and Judith McKay, *When Anger Hurts* (Harbinger Publications, Oakland, Calif., 1989), pp. 46–51.
3. Ibid., p. 11.
4. Ibid., p. 46. Emphasis added.
5. Linda Hanner, John J. Witeck; with Robert B. Clift, *When You're Sick and Don't Know Why* (DCI Publishing, Minneapolis, Minn., 1991), p. 179.
6. Ellen Bass and Laura Davis, *The Courage to Heal* (Harper & Row, Publishers, New York, 1988), p. 203.
7. Deborah Tannen, *You Just Don't Understand* (Random House/Ballantine Books, New York, 1990), p. 15.
8. Samuel Osherson, *Finding Our Fathers* (Random House/Ballantine Books/A Fawcett Columbine Book, New York, 1986), p. 114.
9. Ibid., p. 113.
10. T. MacNab, "Infertility and Men: A Study of Change and Adaptive Choices in the Lives of Involuntarily Childless Men," (doctoral dissertation, Fielding Institute, Berkeley, Calif., 1984), p. 79, cited by Osherson, *Finding Our Fathers*, pp. 114–115.
11. T. MacNab, "Infertility and Men," cited by Aline P. Zoldbrod, *Men, Women and Infertility* (Macmillan Publishing/Lexington Books, New York, 1993), pp. 20–21.
12. John Gray, *Men Are from Mars, Women Are from Venus* (HarperCollins Publishers, New York, 1992), p. 30.
13. These two quotes are from Zoldbrod, *Men, Women and Infertility*, pp. 29 and 28 respectively, citing T. MacNab, "Infertility and Men."
14. T. MacNab, "Infertility and Men," quoted by Osherson, *Finding Our Fathers*, p. 120.
15. Osherson, *Finding Our Fathers*, pp. 129–130.

2 Secondary Infertility

1. Harriet Fishman Simons, *Wanting Another Child* (Simon & Schuster/The Free Press/Lexington Books, New York, 1995), p. 2.
2. Carla Harkness, *The Infertility Book: A Comprehensive Medical and Emotional Guide* (Celestial Arts, Berkeley, Calif., 1992), p. 77.

3. Bob Deits, *Life after Loss* (Fisher Books, Tucson, Ariz., 1992), pp. 67–68.
4. Simons, *Wanting Another Child,* p. 102. Phrases in quotes were taken by Simons from Darrell Sifford, *Only Child: Being One, Loving One, Understanding One, Raising One* (Harper & Row, Publishers, New York, 1989), p. 13.
5. Patricia Irwin Johnston, *Taking Charge of Infertility* (Perspectives Press, Indianapolis, Ind., 1994), p. 237.
6. Linda P. Salzer, *Surviving Infertility* (HarperCollins Publishers/HarperPerennial, New York, 1991), p. 222.
7. Simons, *Wanting Another Child,* p. 79.

3   Communicating Effectively in Crisis

1. C. G. Jung, *The Collected Works of C. G. Jung,* vol. 17 (Bollingen Foundation, Pantheon Books, New York, 1954), p. 193.
2. Deborah Tannen, *You Just Don't Understand* (Random House/Ballantine Books, New York, 1990), pp. 24–25.
3. Ibid, p. 25.
4. John Gray, *Men Are from Mars, Women Are from Venus* (HarperCollins Publishers, New York, 1992), pp. 132–133.
5. Harville Hendrix, *Getting the Love You Want* (HarperCollins Publishers/HarperPerennial, New York, 1988), p. 132.
6. Aaron Beck M., *Love Is Never Enough* (Harper & Row/Perennial Library, New York, 1988), p. 293.
7. The ideas for the section for husbands come from an article written by Dan Clements, "A Process of Understanding for Men," *RESOLVE National Newsletter,* vol. 8, no. 5 (December 1988), p. 3.
8. Hendrix, *Getting the Love You Want,* p. 137.
9. Ibid., pp. 256–257.
10. Ibid., p. 264.
11. Nancy L. Van Pelt, *How to Talk So Your Mate Will Listen* (Fleming H. Revell, Grand Rapids, Mich., 1989), p. 123.
12. The ideas for conflict resolution in the rest of the answer came from pp. 123–152.

4   Family and Friends

1. Judith Viorst, *Necessary Losses* (Random House/Ballantine Books/Fawcett Gold Medal, New York, 1986), p. 187.
2. David Spiegel et al., "Effect of Psychosocial Treatment on Survival of Patients with Metastatic Breast Cancer," *Lancet* (October 14, 1989), pp. 888–891, cited by Tony Schwartz, *What Really Matters* (Bantam Books, New York, 1995), pp. 211–213.
3. David Treadway, *Good Grief,* audiotape of a lecture given at the *Family Therapy Networker* Conference, March 23–26, 1995, Omni Shoreham, Washington, D.C. (produced by The Resource Link, Norcross, Ga.).
4. Merle Bombardieri, *The Baby Decision* (Rawson Wade Publishers, New York, 1981), p. 82.
5. Ibid., pp. 82–91.
6. Vivien Kellerman, "DES Fears Linger Despite Lawsuit," *New York Times* (March 19, 1995), Long Island section, pp. 1 and 6.
7. Gay Becker, *Healing the Infertile Family* (Bantam Books, New York, 1990), p. 129.
8. Robert Veninga, *A Gift of Hope* (Ballantine Books, New York, 1985), pp. 159–160.

9. Viorst, *Necessary Losses*, pp. 197–198.

10. Ibid, p. 197.

6   Dealing with the Medical Community

1. We owe much of the research for this chapter to Susan L. Cooper and Elizabeth S. Glazer, who produced a labor of love and knowledge in their book *Beyond Infertility: The New Paths to Parenthood* (Macmillan Publishing/Lexington Books, New York, 1994). They were the first to discuss in depth the new reproductive technologies from both medical and emotional viewpoints.

2. Diane N. Clapp, *Selecting an Infertility Physician* (RESOLVE National Office, Somerville, Mass., fact sheet no. 16, June 1996), p. 2.

3. Ibid.

4. Grace Moses, "Communicating with Your Physician," *Left Sidelines* (a publication of Sidelines, Laguna Beach, Calif., 1994), pp. 13–14.

5. Adapted from ibid. Some of the wording has been changed to meet the needs of infertility patients.

6. Lauri M. Aesoph, "Using Naturopathic Medicine to Treat Infertility," RESOLVE *National Newsletter,* vol. 18, no. 1 (January 1993), p. 1.

7. Information in this paragraph comes from *Questions to Ask If You Are Seeking Help with Infertility from Alternative Treatment Practioners* (RESOLVE National Office, Somerville, Mass., fact sheet, May 1995), p. 5.

8. Information for this paragraph came from Carla Harkness, *The Infertility Book: A Comprehensive Medical and Emotional Guide* (Celestial Arts, Berkeley, Calif., 1992), p. 239; and Helene S. Rosenberg and Yakov M. Epstein, *Getting Pregnant When You Thought You Couldn't* (Warner Books, New York, 1993), pp. 94–95.

9. Cooper and Glazer, *Beyond Infertility,* p. 309.

10. Ibid., pp. 312–314.

11. Ibid.

12. Coleen Friedman, personal communication, September 1996.

13. Aline P. Zoldbrod, *Men, Women and Infertility* (Macmillan/Lexington Books, New York), p. 203.

14. Sheldon H. Cherry and Carolyn D. Runowicz, *The Menopause Book* (Macmillan Publishing, New York, 1994), p. 22.

7   Working Through Loss

1. Carol Staudacher, *Men & Grief: A Guide for Men Surviving the Death of a Loved One* (New Harbinger Publications, Oakland, Calif., 1991), P. 150. Staudacher's words have been adapted by the authors from prose into poetry.

2. Hope Edelman, *Motherless Daughters: The Legacy of Loss* (Addison Wesley Publishing, Reading, Mass., 1994), pp. 5–6.

3. This list is a distillation of personal experiences, interviews, and all the books we have read relating to loss.

4. Dennis Klass, "Marriage and Divorce among Bereaved Parents in a Self-Help Group" *OMEGA,* vol. 17, no. 3 (Baywood Publishing Co., 1986–1987), p. 239.

5. Alla Renée Bozarth, *Life Is Goodbye, Life Is Hello: Grieving Well through All Kinds of Loss* (CompCare Publishers, Minneapolis, Minn., 1982), p. 25.

6. Carol Staudacher, *Men & Grief* pp. 143–144.

7. Some of the information regarding anniversary reaction is taken from Ingrid Kohn and Perry-Lynn Moffitt, *A Silent Sorrow: Pregnancy Loss, Guidance and Support for You and Your Family* (Dell Publishing/A Delta Book, New York, 1992), p. 21.

8. Richard C. Hall et al., "Grief Following Spontaneous Abortion," *Psychiatric Clinics of North America,* vol. 10, no. 3 (September 1987), p. 408.

9. Regina Sara Ryan, *No Child in My Life* (Stillpoint Publishing, Walpole, N.H., 1993), pp. 68–69.

10. Bozarth, *Life Is Goodbye, Life Is Hello,* p.7.

11. Ibid., p. 5.

12. Carla Harkness, *The Infertility Book: A Comprehensive Medical and Emotional Guide* (Celestial Arts, Berkeley, Calif., 1992), p. 182.

13. General information regarding children's reactions to loss is taken from Kohn and Moffitt, *A Silent Sorrow,* pp. 238–247.

14. David H. Barlow and Michelle G. Craske, *Mastery of Your Anxiety and Panic* (Graywind Publications, Albany, N.Y., 1989), pp. 1–3.

15. Ibid., pp. 1–5.

16. Bozarth, *Life Is Goodbye, Life Is Hello,* pp. 1 and 2 of the Introduction.

8   Religion, Spirituality, Myths, and Miracles

1. We borrowed the idea for this approach from Larry Dossey, *Healing Words: The Power of Prayer and the Practice of Medicine* (HarperCollins, New York, 1993), pp. xiii–xiv.

2. Marianne Williamson, *A Return to Love* (HarperCollins Publishers, New York, 1993), p. 52.

3. Joan Borysenko, *Fire in the Soul: A New Psychology of Spiritual Optimism* (Warner Books, New York, 1993), p. 70.

4. These questions were changed to fit the needs of people experiencing infertility, the original idea came from Aphrodite Matsakis, *I Can't Get Over It: A Handbook for Trauma Survivors* (New Harbinger Publications, Oakland, Calif., 1992), p. 214.

5. Lynda Rutledge Stephenson, *Give Us a Child: Coping with the Personal Crisis of Infertility* (Harper & Row Publishers, San Francisco, 1987), p. 185.

6. Ibid., p. 188.

7. Larry Dossey, *Healing Words,* p. 190, citing Howard Wolinsky, "Prayers Do Aid Sick, Study Finds," *Chicago Sun Times* (January 26, 1986). The study in question is Randolph C. Byrd, "Positive Therapeutic Effects of Intercessory Prayer in a Coronary Care Unit Population," *Southern Medical Journal,* vol. 81, no. 7 (July 1988), pp. 826–829.

8. Reinhold Niebuhr, "Discernment," in Veronica Zundel, ed., *Famous Prayers* (William B. Eerdmans Publishing, Grand Rapids, Mich., 1984), p. 87. Emphasis added.

9. Psalm 139:7–10. Scripture taken from *The Holy Bible, New International Version* (The International Bible Society; Zondervan Bible Publishers, Grand Rapids, Mich., 1984).

10. Michael Gold, *And Hanna Wept: Infertility, Adoption, and the Jewish Couple* (Jewish Publication Society, Philadelphia, 1988), p. 165.

11. Ibid., p. 183.

12. Stephenson, *Give Us a Child,* cited by Dan Morris, "All We Wanted Was a Baby of Our Own," *U.S. Catholic* (February 1992), p. 34.

13. Ideas and quotes in this paragraph come from Arthur Griel, *Not Yet Pregnant* (Rutgers University Press, New Brunswick, N. J., 1991), pp. 172–173.

14. Elizabeth Noble, *Having Your Baby by Donor Insemination* (Houghton-Mifflin, Boston, 1987), p. 210.

15. Donald DeMarco, "There's No Such Thing as a Right to Bear Children," *Sounding Board, U.S. Catholic* (August 1989), p. 18. *Sounding Board* is a publication mailed in advance to *U.S. Catholic* subscribers. *U.S. Catholic* readers' answers to the questions raised in *Sounding Board* are a balanced reflection of their comments about the article as a whole appear in the journal *Feedback.*

16. Morris, "A Baby of Our Own," p. 34.

17. Arthur Griel, *Not Yet Pregnant: Infertile Couples in Contemporary America* (Rutgers University Press, New Brunswick, N.J., 1991), p. 54, citing Melvin Lerner, *The Belief in a Just World* (Plenum Press, New York, 1980).

18. Janet L. Sha, *Mothers of Thyme: Customs and Rituals of Infertility and Miscarriage* (Lida Rose Press, Ann Arbor, Mich., 1990), p. 27.

19. Ibid.

20. Stephenson, *Give Us a Child*, p. 183.

21. Irene Siegel, personal communication, 1995.

22. Louise L. Hay, *Heart Thoughts: A Treasury of Inner Wisdom* (Hay House, Santa Monica, Calif., 1990), p. 206.

23. Ingrid Kohn and Perry-Lynn Moffitt, *A Silent Sorrow: Pregnancy Loss Guidance and Support for You and Your Family* (Dell Publishing/A Delta Book, New York, 1992), p. 185.

24. Vernell Klassen Miller, *Meditations for Adoptive Parents* (Herald Press, Scottdale, Pa., 1992), p. 32.

25. Kohn and Moffitt, *A Silent Sorrow*, pp. 341–345.

26. Marilyn Black Phemister, "Tears in Season," in *The Voice of the Windmill* (Star Books, Wilson, N.C., 1988), p. 92, quoted in Miller, *Meditations for Adoptive Parents*, p. 23.

27. The ideas and concepts for this "Goodbye Service" come from Kohn and Moffitt, *A Silent Sorrow*, pp. 340–365.

9   Decision Making and Infertility

1. Helen Keller, *The Faith of Helen Keller* (Hallmark Cards, Kansas City, 1967).

2. Lynda Rutledge Stephenson, *Give Us a Child: Coping with the Personal Crisis of Infertility* (Harper & Row Publishers, San Francisco, 1987), pp. 194 and 195.

3. John D. Arnold, *Make Up Your Mind!* (Amacom/A Division of American Management Associations, New York, 1978), pp. 114.

4. Alexandra Stoddard, *Making Choices* (William Morrow & Company, New York, 1994), p. 21.

5. Susan Jeffers, *Feel the Fear and Do It Anyway* (Harcourt Brace Jovanovich Publishers, San Diego, 1987), pp. 33–46.

6. Ibid.

7. Many of the ideas and phrases in the following answer are taken from Jean Carter and Mike Carter, *Sweet Grapes: How to Stop Being Infertile and Start Living Again* (Perspectives Press, Indianapolis, Ind., 1989), pp. 80–85.

8. Merle Bombardieri, *Childfree Decision-Making* (RESOLVE national office, fact sheet #5, 1995), p. 4.

9. Carla Harkness, *The Infertility Book: A Comprehensive Medical and Emotional Guide* (Celestial Arts, Berkeley, Calif., 1992), p. 218.

10. Aaron Britvan, Review of *Adoption Law and Practice* by Joan Hollinger and 13 other contributing authors, *Family Advocate* (American Bar Association, Chicago), vol. XII, no. 2 (Fall 1989), p. 7.

10   Child-Free Living

1. Louis Untermeyer, ed., *The Road Not Taken: An Introduction to Robert Frost* (Holt, Rinehart & Winston, New York, 1962), p. 271.

2. Amara Bachu, *Fertility of American Women: June 1994* (U.S. Bureau of the Census, Current Population Reports P20-482, U.S. Government Printing Office, Washington, D.C., 1995) Table F; also personal communication with Amara Bachu, March 11, 1997.

3. Clarissa Pinkola Estés, *Women Who Run with the Wolves: Myths and Stories of the Wild Woman Archetype* (Random House/Ballantine Books, New York, 1992), p. 181.

4. *American Heritage Dictionary,* 3rd ed.; s.v. "-less" and "-free."

5. Jean Carter and Mike Carter, *Sweet Grapes: How to Stop Being Infertile and Start Living Again* (Perspectives Press, Indianapolis, Ind., 1989), p. 114.

6. Bachu, *Fertility of American Women,* Table F.

7. Linda Hunt Anton, *Never to Be a Mother: A Guide for All Women Who Didn't—Or Couldn't—Have Children* (HarperCollins Publishers, New York, 1992), pp. 179–185.

8. Carter and Carter, *Sweet Grapes,* p. 57.

9. The following description of the self-empowerment process is from Marcia Chellis, *Ordinary Women, Extraordinary Lives* (Penguin Books/Viking Penguin, New York, 1992), pp. 1–22.

10. For more in-depth information, see Susan Lang in *Women without Children: The Reasons, the Rewards, the Regrets* (Pharos Books, New York, 1991), pp. 222–223. Lang cites several studies: Karen Peterson, Gannett News Service, "Study: When Kids Leave Home, Parents' Marriage Gets Better," *Ithaca Journal* (August 22, 1990); Karen Polonko et al., "Childlessness and Marital Satisfaction," *Journal of Family Issues,* vol. 3, no. 4 (December 1982), pp. 545–573; and Karen S. Renne, "Childlessness, Health and Marital Satisfaction," *Social Biology,* vol. 23, no. 3 (1976), p. 196.

11. Lang, *Women without Children,* p. 223, citing Victor Callan, "The Personal and Marital Adjustments of Mothers and of Voluntarily and Involuntarily Childless Wives," *Journal of Marriage and the Family,* vol. 49 (November 1987), pp. 847–856.

12. Ibid., pp. 241, 243.

13. Carter and Carter, *Sweet Grapes,* p. 114.

14. Anton, *Never to Be a Mother,* p. 107.

11   Waiting for Your Baby

1. Aaron Britvan, personal communication, October 1995.

2. Carlos Castaneda, *The Teachings of Don Juan: A Yaqui Way of Knowledge* (University of California Press, Berkeley, 1968), p. 76.

3. Amy Rackear, "In Our Own Backyard: For Love of Adam," *RESOLVE of New York City Newsletter* (June 1994), p. 9.

4. Ibid, p. 7.

5. N.Y. State Adoptive Parents Committee, "Positive Adoption Language," *ADOPTALK* (April 1994), p. 9.

6. Peter Benson, Anu Sharma, and Eugene Roehlkepartain, *Growing Up Adopted* (Search Institute, Minneapolis, Minn., 1994), p. 50; quoting David Brodzinsky, "A Stress and Coping Model of Adoption Adjustment," in D. M. Brodzinsky and M. D. Schechter, eds., *The Psychology of Adoption* (Oxford University Press, New York, 1990), pp. 3–24.

7. Benson et al., *Growing Up Adopted,* p. 50.

8. Miriam Komar, *Communicating with the Adopted Child* (Walker & Company, New York, 1991), pp. 27–28.

9. Ellen Sarasohn Glazer, *The Long Awaited Stork* (Macmillan Publishing/Lexington Books, Lexington, Mass., 1990), p. 20.

10. Aline P. Zoldbrod, *Men, Women and Infertility* (Macmillan Publishing/Lexington Books, New York, 1993), p. 59.

11. Ibid., pp. 163–164.

12. Candace Hurley, personal communication, August 1995.

13. Susan L. Cooper and Ellen S. Glazer, *Beyond Infertility: The New Paths to Parenthood* (Macmillan Publishing/Lexington Books, New York, 1994), p. 108.

14. The information in this answer regarding the work of Mary McKinney, Ph.D., comes from personal communication, March 1997, as well as from her article "Emotional Effects of Selective Pregnancy Reduction," *RESOLVE of Long Island Newsletter* (Winter 1995), pp. 12–14.

15. Rochelle Friedman and Bonnie Gradstein, *Surviving Pregnancy Loss* (Little, Brown, Boston, Mass., 1992), p. 120.

16. Maureen Boyle, personal communication, August 1995.

17. McKinney, "Emotional Aspects of Selective Pregnancy Reduction," p. 13.

Part IV   Epilogue

1. Aline P. Zoldbrod, *Men, Women and Infertility* (Macmillan/Lexington Books, New York, 1993), pp. 177–178, quoting Seymour Fisher, *Sexual Images of the Self: The Psychology of Erotic Sensations and Illusion* (Lawrence Erlbaum Associates, Hillsdale, N.J., 1989), pp. 263 and 266.

2. Hope Edelman, *Motherless Daughters: The Legacy of Loss* (Addison-Wesley Publishing, Reading, Mass., 1994), pp. 279–280.

Part V   Treating Infertility: A Guide for Professionals

1. Randi Guggenheimer, personal interview, 1996.

2. Ibid.

3. Sonia Hieger, "The Treatment of Infertile Clients" (paper submitted to the authors, 1995), pp. 1–2.

4. Diagnoses listed from *Diagnostic Criteria from DSM IV™* (American Psychiatric Association, Washington, D.C., 1994), pp. 274 and 279.

5. This quote, and the quotes and discussion in the following paragraphs about Gestalt therapy, are drawn from Joyce Magid, "A Gestalt Therapy Approach to Infertility" (paper submitted to the authors, 1995), pp. 3–4.

6. The quotes in this paragraph are from Susan Gardner, "Psychotherapy and Infertility" (paper submitted to the authors, 1995), pp. 1–2.

7. Magid, "A Gestalt Therapy Approach," p. 1.

8. Ibid., p. 4.

9. Nancy Newman, "Application of Family Systems Concepts in Infertility," paper presented to Advanced Course in Infertility Counseling: Ethical Dilemmas and Therapeutic Interventions (American Society of Reproductive Medicine, Orlando, Fla., April 1994), and personal communications, September 1995 and March 1997.

10. The ideas and quote in this paragraph come from David P. Eckert, "Men and Infertility" (paper submitted to the authors, 1995), p. 1.

11. Ira Kalina, "Marital Therapy with an Infertile Couple" (paper submitted to the authors, 1995), p. 3.

12. Ibid.

13. Linda Salzer, "Information for Professionals" (paper submitted to the authors, 1995), p. 1.

14. Sonia Hieger, "Love, Sex, Romance and Infertility," *RESOLVE of Long Island Newsletter* (March 1996), p. 4.

15. Hieger, "The Treatment of Infertile Clients," p. 1.

16. Newman, "Application of Family Systems Concepts," p. 10.

17. Ideas in this section come from Gardner, "Psychotherapy and Infertility."

18. Ibid., p. 2.
19. The ideas in this section are drawn from Sheryl Stern, "Art Therapy and Infertility Support Groups" (paper submitted to the authors, 1995).
20. All the quotes, and much of the material presented from here to the end of this answer, are from Dominic Candido and Teresa Candido, "Cognitive Therapy and Infertility: A Crisis of Purpose" (paper submitted to the authors, 1995), pp. 1–5.
21. Alice D. Domar, "Stress and Infertility in Women," in Sandra R. Lieblum, ed., *Infertility: Psychological Issues and Counseling Strategies* (John Wiley & Sons, New York, 1997), p. 67.
22. Ibid., p. 70.
23. Ibid., p. 81.
24. Sybil Lefferts, "The Mind/Body Connection and Infertility" (paper submitted to the authors, 1995), p. 2.
25. Peggy Bruhn, "Loss and Infertility" (paper submitted to the authors, 1995), p. 1.
26. Lefferts, "The Mind/Body Connection," p. 2.
27. Personal communication with Harry Rieckelman, director, and Fr. Paul Costello, director of research, both for the Institute for Narrative Therapy in Washington, D.C., July 1995.
28. Patricia Kelley, "Narrative Theory and Social Work Treatment," in Francis J. Turner, ed., *Social Work Treatment: Interlocking Theoretical Approaches,* 4th ed. (The Free Press, New York, 1996), p. 462.
29. Ibid., p. 463.
30. Bill O'Hanolan, "The Third Wave," *The Family Therapy Networker,* vol. 18, no. 6 (November/December 1994), p. 24.
31. The story about this woman's adoption loss, described and quoted here in some detail, is taken from a personal interview with Rieckelman and Costello, July 1995.
32. Mary Sykes Wylie, "Panning for Gold," *The Family Therapy Networker,* vol. 18, no. 6 (November/December 1994), p. 43.
33. This quote and the following quotes and discussion on dream work, creative expression, and imagery drawn from Alla Renée Bozarth, "Soul Work with the Infertile Client" (paper submitted to the authors, 1995), pp. 1–2.
34. Roger J. Woolger *Other Lives, Other Selves: A Jungian Psychotherapist Discovers Past Lives* (Bantam Books, New York, 1988), pp. 33–34.
35. Ibid., p. 82.
36. Lefferts, "The Mind/Body Connection" pp. 4–6.
37. Aline P. Zoldbrod, *Men, Women and Infertility* (Macmillan Publishing/Lexington Books, New York, 1993), p. 203.
38. Magid, "A Gestalt Therapy Approach," pp. 2 and 3.

Appendix I   Self-Help Guide

1. Herbert Benson and Eileen M. Stuart, *The Wellness Book* (Birch Lane Press, Carol Publishing Group, New York, 1992), pp. 42–43.
2. Aline P. Zoldbrod, *Getting Around the Boulder in the Road: Using Imagery to Cope with Fertility Problems* (Center for Reproductive Problems, Lexington, Mass., 1990), pp. 6–13.
3. Ibid., p. 11.
4. Adapted from Belleruth Naparstek, *Staying Well with Guided Imagery* (Warner Books, New York, 1994), pp. 76–79.
5. Alice Domar and Henry Dreher, *Healing Mind, Healthy Woman: Using the Mind-Body Connection to Manage Stress and Take Control of Your Life* (Henry Holt, New York, 1996), p. 56.
6. Ibid.

REFERENCES AND SUGGESTED READINGS

1 Who Am I?

Bass, Ellen, and Laura Davis. *The Courage to Heal.* Harper & Row/Perennial Library, New York, 1988.

Cherry, Sheldon H., and Carolyn D. Runowicz. *The Menopause Book.* Macmillan Publishing, New York, 1994.

Deits, Bob. *Life after Loss.* Fisher Books, Tucson, Ariz., 1992.

Gray, John. *Men Are from Mars, Women Are from Venus.* HarperCollins Publishers, New York, 1992.

Greenberg, Jay R., and Stephen A. Mitchell. *Object Relations in Psychoanalytic Theory.* Harvard University Press, Cambridge, Mass., 1993.

Hanner, Linda, and John J. Witeck; with Rober B. Clift. *When You're Sick and Don't Know Why.* DCI Publishing, Minneapolis, Minn., 1991.

Josselson, Ruthellen. *Finding Herself.* Jossey-Bass Publishers, San Francisco, 1987.

MacNab, T. "Infertility and Men: A Study of Change and Adaptive Choices in the Lives of Involuntarily Childless Men." Doctoral dissertation, Fielding Institute, Berkeley, Calif., 1984.

McKay, Matthew, Peter D. Rogers, and Judith McKay. *When Anger Hurts.* New Harbinger Publications, Oakland, Calif., 1989.

Osherson, Samuel. *Finding Our Fathers.* Random House/Ballantine Books/A Fawcett Columbine Book, New York, 1986.

Tannen, Deborah. *You Just Don't Understand.* Random House/Ballantine Books, New York, 1990.

Zoldbrod, Aline P. *Men, Women and Infertility.* Macmillan Publishing/Lexington Books, New York, 1993.

2 Secondary Infertility

Deits, Bob. *Life after Loss.* Fisher Books, Tucson, Ariz., 1992.

Harkness, Carla. *The Infertility Book: A Comprehensive Medical and Emotional Guide.* Celestial Arts, Berkeley, Calif., 1992.

Johnston, Patricia Irwin. *Taking Charge of Infertility.* Perspectives Press, Indianapolis, Ind., 1994.

Salzer, Linda P. *Surviving Infertility.* HarperCollins Publishers/HarperPerennial, New York, 1991.

Sifford, Darrell. *Only Child: Being One, Loving One, Understanding One, Raising One.* Harper & Row, Publishers, New York, 1989.

Simons, Harriet Fishman. *Wanting Another Child.* Simon & Shuster/The Free Press/Lexington Books, New York, 1995.

3 Communicating Effectively in Crisis

Barreca, Regina. *Perfect Husbands.* Random House, New York, 1993.

Beck, Aaron. *Love Is Never Enough.* Harper & Row/Perennial Library, New York, 1988.

Clements, Dan. "A Process of Understanding for Men," *RESOLVE National Newsletter,* vol. 8, no. 5 (December 1988), pp. 3–4.

Gray, John. *Men Are from Mars, Women Are from Venus.* HarperCollins Publishers, New York, 1992.

Hendrix, Harville. *Getting the Love You Want: A Guide for Couples.* HarperCollins Publishers/Harper-Perennial, New York, 1988.

Jung, C. G. *The Collected Works of C. G. Jung.* Vol. 17. Bollingen Foundation, Pantheon Books, New York, 1954.

Notarius, Clifford, and Howard Markman. *We Can Work It Out.* G. P. Putman's Sons, New York, 1993.

Tannen, Deborah. *That's Not What I Meant.* Random House/Ballantine Books, New York, 1986.

Tannen, Deborah. *You Just Don't Understand.* Random House/Ballantine Books, New York, 1990.

Van Pelt, Nancy L. *How to Talk So Your Mate Will Listen.* Fleming H. Revell, Grand Rapids, Mich., 1989.

Wallerstein, Judith S., and Sandra Blakeslee. *The Good Marriage.* Houghton-Mifflin, Boston, 1995.

4 Family and Friends

Becker, Gay. *Healing the Infertile Family.* Bantam Books, New York, 1990.

Bombardieri, Merle. *The Baby Decision.* Rawson, Wade Publishers, New York, 1981.

Burke, Ronald. "Support Groups Aid in Achieving Pregnancy," *RESOLVE National Newsletter,* vol. 16, no. 5 (December 1991).

Burns, David. *The Feeling Good Handbook.* Plume Books, New York, 1989.

Fishel, Elizabeth. *Sisters.* William Morrow, New York, 1979.

Griel, Arthur L. *Not Yet Pregnant: Infertile Couples in Contemporary America.* Rutgers University Press, New Brunswick, N.J., 1991.

Jeffers, Susan. *Dare to Connect.* Random House/Ballantine Books/A Fawcett Columbine Book, New York, 1992.

Kellerman, Vivien. "DES Fears Linger Despite Lawsuit," *New York Times* (March 19, 1995), Long Island section, pp. 1 and 6.

Salzer, Linda. *Surviving Infertility.* HarperCollins Publishers/HarperPerennial, New York, 1991.

Schwartz, Tony. *What Really Matters.* Bantam Books, New York, 1995.

Spiegel, David, et al. "Effect of Psychosocial Treatment on Survival of Patients with Metastatic Breast Cancer," *Lancet* (October 14, 1989), pp. 888–891.

Treadway, David. *Good Grief.* Audiotape of a lecture given at the *Family Therapy Networker* Conference, March 23–26, 1995, Omni Shoreham, Washington, D.C. Produced by The Resource Link, Norcross, Ga.

Veninga, Robert. *A Gift of Hope.* Ballantine Books, New York, 1985.

Viorst, Judith. *Necessary Losses.* Random House/Ballantine Books/Fawcett Gold Medal, New York, 1986.

6 Dealing with the Medical Community

Aesoph, Lauri M. "Using Naturopathic Medicine to Treat Infertility," *RESOLVE National Newsletter,* vol. 18, no. 1 (January 1993), pp. 1 and 4.

Andrews, Lori. *Between Strangers: Surrogate Mothers.* Harper & Row, New York, 1989.

Berger, Gary, Marc Goldstein, and Mark Fuerst. *The Couples Guide to Fertility.* Doubleday, New York, 1995.

Boston Women's Collective. *The New Our Bodies Ourselves.* Simon & Schuster, New York, 1985.

Cherry, Sheldon H., and Carolyn D. Runowicz. *The Menopause Book.* Macmillan Publishing, New York, 1994.

Clapp, Diane. *Selecting an Infertility Physician.* RESOLVE National Office, Somerville, Mass., fact sheet no. 16, June 1996.

Cooper, Susan L., and Ellen S. Glazer. *Beyond Infertility: The New Paths to Parenthood.* Macmillan Publishing/Lexington Books, New York, 1994.

Harkness, Carla. *The Infertility Book: A Comprehensive Medical and Emotional Guide.* Celestial Arts, San Francisco, 1992.

Noble, Elizabeth. *Having Your Baby by Donor Insemination: A Complete Resource Guide.* Houghton-Mifflin, Boston, 1987.

Marrs, Richard. *Dr. Marrs' Fertility Book.* Delacorte Press, New York, 1997.

Menning, Barbara Eck. *Infertility: A Guide for Childless Couples.* Prentice-Hall, Englewood Cliffs, N.J., 1988.

Moses, Grace. "Communicating with Your Physician," *Left Sidelines* (a publication of Sidelines, Laguna Beach, Calif., 1994), pp. 13–15.

Raab, Diana. *Getting Pregnant and Staying Pregnant.* Hunter House, Claremont, Calif., 1991.

Rosenberg, Helene S., and Yakov M. Epstein. *Getting Pregnant When You Thought You Couldn't.* Warner Books, New York, 1993.

Savage, Judith A. *Mourning Unlived Lives: A Psychological Study of Childbearing Loss.* Chiron Publications, Wilmette, Ill., 1989.

Scher, Jonathan. *Preventing Miscarriage: The Good News.* Harper & Row Publishers, New York, 1990.

Shapiro, Constance Hoenk. *Infertility and Pregnancy Loss: A Guide for Helping Professionals.* Jossey-Bass Publishers, San Francisco, 1988.

Zoldbrod, Aline P. *Men, Women and Infertility,* Macmillan Publishing/Lexington Books, New York, 1993.

7   Working Through Loss

Barlow, David H., and Michelle G. Craske. *Mastery of Your Anxiety and Panic.* Graywind Publications, Albany, N.Y., 1989.

Bozarth, Alla Renée. *Life Is Goodbye, Life Is Hello: Grieving Well through All Kinds of Loss.* CompCare Publishers, Minneapolis, Minn., 1982.

Conway, Patricia, and Deborah Valentine. "Reproductive Losses and Grieving," in *Infertility and Adoption: A Guide for Social Work Practice.* Haworth Press, Binghamton, N.Y., 1988, pp. 43–64.

Davis, Deborah L. *Empty Cradle, Broken Heart.* Fulcrum Publishing, Golden, Colo., 1991.

Deits, Bob. *Life after Loss.* Fisher Books, Tucson, Ariz., 1992.

Edelman, Hope. *Motherless Daughters: The Legacy of Loss.* Addison-Wesley Publishing, Reading, Mass., 1994.

Fletcher, John C., and Mark I. Evans. "Maternal Bonding in Early Fetal Ultrasound Examination," *New England Journal of Medicine,* vol. 308, no. 7 (February 17, 1983), pp. 392–393.

Freese, Arthur. *Help for Your Grief.* Schocken Books, New York, 1977.

Friedman, Rochelle, and Bonnie Gradstein. *Surviving Pregnancy Loss.* Little, Brown, Boston, 1992.

Hall, Richard C., Thomas P. Beresford, and Jose E. Quinones. "Grief Following Spontaneous Abortion," *Psychiatric Clinics of North America,* vol. 10, no. 3 (September 1987), pp. 405–420.

Harkness, Carla. *The Infertility Book: A Comprehensive Medical and Emotional Guide.* Celestial Arts, Berkeley, Calif., 1992.

Ilse, Sherokee. *Empty Arms.* Wintergreen Press, Maple Plain, Minn., 1990.

Kennell, John H., Howard Slyter, and Marshall H. Klaus. "The Mourning Response of Parents to the Death of a Newborn Infant," *New England Journal of Medicine,* vol. 283, no. 7 (August 13, 1970), pp. 344–349.

Klass, Dennis. "Marriage and Divorce among Bereaved Parents in a Self-Help Group," *OMEGA,* vol. 17, no. 3 (Baywood Publishing, 1986–1987), pp. 237–249.

Kohn, Ingrid, and Perry-Lynn Moffitt. *A Silent Sorrow: Pregnancy Loss, Guidance and Support for You and Your Family.* Dell Publishing/A Delta Book, New York, 1992.

Matsakis, Aphrodite. *I Can't Get Over It: A Handbook for Trauma Survivors.* New Harbinger Publications, Oakland, Calif., 1992.

Raphael, Beverly. *The Anatomy of Bereavement.* Basic Books, New York, 1993.

Ryan, Regina Sara. *No Child in My Life.* Stillpoint Publishing, Walpole, N.H., 1993.

Slaby, Andrew E. *Aftershock.* Villard Books, New York, 1989.

Staudacher, Carol. *Men & Grief: A Guide for Men Surviving the Death of a Loved One.* New Harbinger Publications, Oakland, Calif., 1991.

8   Religion, Spirituality, Myths, and Miracles

Borysenko, Joan. *Fire in the Soul: A New Psychology of Spiritual Optimism.* Warner Books, New York, 1993.

Byrd, Randolph C. "Positive Therapeutic Effects of Intercessory Prayer in a Coronary Care Unit Population," *Southern Medical Journal,* vol. 81, no. 7 (July 1988), pp. 826–829.

Chopra, Deepak. *Ageless Body, Timeless Mind.* Harmony Books, New York, 1993.

DeMarco, Donald. "There's No Such Thing as a Right to Bear Children," *Sounding Board, U.S. Catholic* (August 1989), pp. 13–19.

Dossey, Larry. *Healing Words: The Power of Prayer and the Practice of Medicine.* HarperCollins, New York, 1993.

Gold, Michael. *And Hannah Wept: Infertility, Adoption, and the Jewish Couple.* Jewish Publication Society, Philadelphia, 1988.

Griel, Arthur L. *Not Yet Pregnant: Infertile Couples in Contemporary America.* Rutgers University Press, Brunswick, N.J., 1991.

Hay, Louise. *Heart Thoughts: A Treasury of Inner Wisdom.* Hay House, Santa Monica, Calif., 1990.

Hull, Richard T. *Ethical Issues in the New Reproductive Technologies.* Wadsworth Publishing, Belmont, Calif., 1990.

The Holy Bible, New International Version. The International Bible Society, Zondervan Bible Publishers, Grand Rapids, Mich., 1984.

Klein, Charles. *How to Forgive When You Can't Forget: Healing Our Personal Relationships.* Liebling Press, Bellmore, N.Y., 1995.

Kohn, Ingrid, and Perry-Lynn Moffitt. *A Silent Sorrow: Pregnancy Loss, Guidance and Support for You and Your Family.* Dell Publishing/A Delta Book, New York, 1992.

Kushner, Harold. *How Good Do We Have to Be?* Little, Brown, Boston, 1996.

Kushner, Harold. *When Bad Things Happen to Good People.* Schocken Books, New York, 1981.

Kushner, Harold. *Who Needs God.* Summit Books, New York, 1989.

Larson, Bob. *Straight Answers on the New Age.* Thomas Nelson Publishers, Nashville, Tenn., 1989.

Matsakis, Aphrodite. *I Can't Get Over It: A Handbook for Trauma Survivors.* New Harbinger Publications, Oakland, Calif., 1992.

Miller, Vernell Klassen. *Meditations for Adoptive Parents.* Herald Press, Scottdale, Pa., 1992.

Moore, Thomas. *Care of the Soul.* HarperPerennial, New York, 1992.

Morris, Dan. "All We Wanted Was a Baby of Our Own," *U.S. Catholic* (February 1992), pp. 28–35.

Noble, Elizabeth. *Having Your Baby by Donor Insemination: A Complete Resource Guide.* Houghton-Mifflin, Boston, 1987.

Phemister, Marilyn Black. *The Voice of the Windmill.* Star Books, Wilson, N.C., 1988.

Ryan, Regina Sara. *No Child in My Life.* Stillpoint Publishing, Walpole, N.H., 1993.

Savage, Judith A. *Mourning Unlived Lives: A Psychological Study of Childbearing Loss.* Chiron Publications, Wilmette, Ill., 1989.

Sha, Janet L. *Mother of Thyme: Customs and Rituals of Infertility and Miscarriage.* Lida Rose Press, Ann Arbor, Mich., 1990.

Siegel, Bernie S. *Peace, Love and Healing.* HarperPerennial, New York, 1990.

Sowers, Meredith L. Young. *Spiritual Crisis.* Stillpoint Publishing, Walpole, N.H., 1993.

Stephenson, Lynda Rutledge. *Give Us a Child: Coping with the Personal Crisis of Infertility.* Harper & Row, Publishers, New York, 1987.

Williamson, Marianne. *A Return to Love.* HarperCollins Publishers, New York, 1993.

Wolinsky, Howard. "Prayers Do Aid Sick, Study Finds," *Chicago Sun Times* (January 26, 1986), p. 30.

Zundel, Veronica, ed. *Famous Prayers.* William B. Eerdmans Publishing, Grand Rapids, Mich., 1984.

9   Decision Making and Infertility . . .

Arnold, John D. *Make Up Your Mind!* Amacon, New York, 1978.

Bass, Ellen, and Laura Davis. *The Courage to Heal.* Harper & Row/Perennial Library, New York, 1988.

Becker, Gay. *Healing the Infertile Family.* Bantam Books, New York, 1990.

Bombardieri, Merle. *The Baby Decision.* Rawson Wade Publishers, New York, 1981.

Bombardieri, Merle. *Childfree Decision-Making.* (*RESOLVE* National Office, Washington, D.C., fact sheet no. 5, 1995).

Carter, Jean W., and Michael Carter. *Sweet Grapes: How to Stop Being Infertile and Start Living Again.* Perspectives Press, Indianapolis, Ind., 1989.

Deits, Bob. *Life after Loss.* Fisher Books, Tucson, Ariz., 1992.

Finley, Guy. *The Secret of Letting Go.* Llewellyn Press, St. Paul, Minn., 1993.

Harkness, Carla. *The Infertility Book: A Comprehensive Medical and Emotional Guide.* Celestial Arts, Berkeley, Calif., 1992.

Jampolsky, Gerald G., and Diane V. Cirincione. *Change Your Mind, Change Your Life.* Bantam Books, New York, 1993.

Jeffers, Susan. *Feel the Fear and Do It Anyway.* Random House/Ballantine Books/A Fawcett Columbine Book, New York, 1987.

Shapiro, Constance Hoenk. *When Part of the Self Is Lost.* Jossey-Bass Publishers, San Francisco, 1993.

Stephenson, Lynda Rutledge. *Give Us a Child: Coping with the Personal Crisis of Infertility.* Harper & Row Publishers, New York, 1987.

Stanton, Annette, and Christine Dunkel Schetter. *Infertility.* Plenum Press, New York, 1991.

Stoddard, Alexandra. *Making Choices.* William Morrow, New York, 1994.

Viscott, David. *Risking.* Pocket Books, New York, 1977.

10   Child-Free Living

Anton, Linda Hunt. *Never to Be a Mother: A Guide for All Women Who Didn't—Or Couldn't—Have Children.* HarperCollins Publishers, New York, 1992.

Bachu, Amaru. *Fertility of American Women: June 1994.* U.S. Bureau of the Census, Current Population Reports P20-482. U.S. Government Printing Office, Washington, D.C., 1995.

Bolles, Richard Nelson. *What Color Is Your Parachute.* Ten Speed Press, Berkeley, Calif., 1996.

Carter, Jean, and Mike Carter. *Sweet Grapes: How to Stop Being Infertile and Start Living Again.* Perspectives Press, Indianapolis, Ind., 1989.

Chellis, Marcia. *Ordinary Women, Extraordinary Lives.* Penguin Books/Viking Penguin, New York, 1992.

Cooney, Barbara. *Miss Rumphius.* Viking Penguin/Puffin Books, New York, 1982.

Estés, Clarissa Pinkola. *Women Who Run with the Wolves: Myths and Stories of the Wild Woman Archetype.* Random House/Ballantine Books, New York, 1992.

Ireland, Mandy S. *Reconceiving Women.* The Guilford Press, New York, 1993.

Lang, Susan. *Women without Children: The Reasons, the Rewards, the Regrets.* Pharos Books, New York, 1991.

May, Elaine Tyler. *Barren in the Promised Land.* HarperCollins/Basic Books, New York, 1995.

Peck, M. Scott. *The Road Less Traveled.* Simon & Schuster/Touchtone Books, New York, 1978.
Untermeyer, Louis, ed. *The Road Not Taken: An Introduction to Robert Frost.* Holt, Rinehart & Winston, New York, 1962.

11   Waiting for Your Baby

Bartholet, Elizabeth. *Family Bonds: Adoption and the Politics of Parenting.* Houghton-Mifflin, Boston, 1993.

Becker, Gay. *Healing the Infertile Family.* Bantam Books, New York, 1990.

Benson, Peter, Anu Sharma, and Eugene Roehlkepartain. *Growing Up Adopted.* Search Institute, Minneapolis, Minn. 1994.

Berends, Polly Berrien. *Whole Child/Whole Parent.* Harper & Row/Perennial Library, New York, 1987.

Castaneda, Carlos. *The Teachings of Don Juan: A Yaqui Way of Knowledge.* University of California Press, Berkeley, 1968.

Cooper, Susan L., and Ellen S. Glazer. *Beyond Infertility: The New Paths to Parenthood.* Macmillan Publishing/Lexington Books, New York, 1994.

Friedman, Rochelle, and Bonnie Gradstein. *Surviving Pregnancy Loss.* Little, Brown, Boston, 1992.

Glazer, Ellen Sarasohn. *The Long Awaited Stork.* Macmillan Publishing/Lexington Books, Lexington, Mass., 1990.

Johnston, Patricia Irwin. *Taking Charge of Infertility.* Perspectives Press, Indianapolis, Ind., 1994.

Komar, Miriam. *Communicating with the Adopted Child.* Walker & Company, New York, 1991.

McKinney, Mary. "Emotional Effects of Selective Pregnancy Reduction," *RESOLVE of Long Island Newsletter* (Winter 1995), pp. 12–14.

Melina, Louis Ruskai. *Raising Adopted Children.* Harper & Row/A Soltice Press Book, New York, 1986.

New York State Adoptive Parents Committee. "Positive Adoption Language," *ADOPTALK* (newsletter; April 1994), p. 9.

Rackear, Amy. "In Our Own Backyard: For the Love of Adam," *RESOLVE of New York City Newsletter* (June 1994), pp. 7–9.

Rosenberg, Elinor. *The Adoption Life Cycle.* The Free Press, New York, 1992.

Ryan, Regina Sara. *No Child in My Life.* Stillpoint Publishing, Walpole, N.H., 1993.

Schwartz, Tony. *What Really Matters.* Bantam Books, New York, 1995.

Sheehy, Gail. *New Passages.* Random House, New York, 1995.

Weingarten, Kathy. *The Mother's Voice.* Harcourt Brace, New York, 1994.

Zoldbrod, Aline P. *Getting Around the Boulder in the Road: Using Imagery to Cope with Fertility Problems.* Center for Reproductive Problems, Lexington, Mass., 1990.

Zoldbrod, Aline P. *Men, Women and Infertility.* Macmillan Publishing/Lexington Books, New York, 1993.

Part IV   Epilogue

Edelman, Hope. *Motherless Daughters: The Legacy of Loss.* Addison-Wesley Publishing, Reading, Mass., 1994.

Fisher, Seymour. *Sexual Images of the Self: The Psychology of Erotic Sensations and Illusion.* Lawrence Erlbaum Associates, Hillsdale, N.J., 1989.

Zoldbrod, Aline P. *Men, Women and Infertility.* Macmillan Publishing/Lexington Books, New York, 1993.

Part V   Treating Infertility: A Guide for Professionals

Beck, Aaron. *Cognitive Therapy of Depression.* The Guilford Press, New York, 1989.

Beck, Judith S. *Cognitive Therapy: Basics and Beyond.* The Guilford Press, New York, 1995.

Benson, Herbert, and Miriam Klipper. *The Relaxation Response.* Avon Books, New York, 1995.

Borysenko, Joan. *Minding the Body, Mending the Mind.* Bantam Books, New York, 1988.

Diagnostic Criteria from DSM IV.™ American Psychiatric Association, Washington, D.C., 1994.

Domar, Alice. *Healing Mind, Healthy Woman: Using the Mind-Body Connection to Manage Stress and Take Control of Your Life.* Henry Holt, New York, 1996.

Domar, Alice. "Stress and Infertility in Women," in Sandra R. Lieblum, ed., *Infertility: Psychological Issues and Counseling Strategies.* John Wiley & Sons, New York, 1997, pp. 67–83.

Elias, Jason, and Katherine Ketcham. *In the House of the Moon: Reclaiming the Feminine Spirit of Healing.* Warner Books, New York, 1995.

Griel, Arthur L. *Not Yet Pregnant: Infertile Couples in Contemporary America.* Rutgers University Press, New Brunswick, N.J., 1991.

Hendrix, Harville. *Getting the Love You Want: A Guide for Couples.* HarperCollins Publishers/HarperPerennial, New York, 1988.

Hermans, Hubert, and Els Hermans-Jansen. *Self Narratives: The Construction of Meaning in Psychotherapy.* The Guilford Press, New York, 1995.

Hieger, Sonia. "Love, Sex, Romance and Infertility," *RESOLVE of Long Island Newsletter* (March 1996), p. 4.

Kabat-Zinn, Jon. *Full Catastrophe Living: Using the Wisdom of Your Body and Mind to Face Stress, Pain and Illness.* Delacorte Press, New York, 1991.

Kelley, Patricia. "Narrative Theory and Social Work Treatment," in Francis J. Turner, ed., *Social Work Treatment: Interlocking Theoretical Approaches,* 4th led. The Free Press, New York, 1996, pp. 461–479.

Lieblum, Sandra R. *Infertility: Psychological Issues and Counseling Strategies.* John Wiley & Sons, New York, 1997.

McGoldrick, Monica, and Candy Gerson. *Genograms in Family Assessment.* W. W. Norton & Company, New York, 1995.

Naparstek, Belleruth. *Staying Well with Guided Imagery.* Warner Books, New York, 1994. (Audiotape series available from Image Paths, 800-800-8661.)

Newman, Nancy. "Application of Family Systems Concepts in Infertility," paper presented to Advanced Course in Infertility Counseling: Ethical Dilemmas and Therapeutic Interventions. American Society for Reproductive Medicine, Orlando, Fla., April 1994.

O'Hanolan, Bill. "The Third Wave," *The Family Therapy Networker,* vol. 18, no. 6. (November/December, 1994), pp. 00–00.

Parry, Alan, and Robert E. Doan. *Story Revisions: Narrative Therapy in the Postmodern World.* The Guilford Press, New York, 1994.

Perls, Federick. *Ego, Hunger and Aggression.* Random House, New York, 1969.

Perls, Federick, Ralph Hefferline, and Paul Goodman. *Gestalt Therapy.* The Gestalt Journal Press, Highland, N.Y., 1994.

Turner, Francis J. *Social Work Treatment: Interlocking Theoretical Approaches.* 4th edition. The Free Press, New York, 1996.

Weiss, Brian. *Many Lives, Many Masters.* Simon & Shuster, New York, 1988.

White, Michael, and David Epston. *Narrative Means to Therapeutic Ends.* W. W. Norton, New York, 1990.

Woolger, Roger J. *Other Lives, Other Selves: A Jungian Psychotherapist Discovers Past Lives.* Bantam Books, New York, 1988.

Wylie, Mary Sykes. "Panning for Gold," *The Family Therapy Networker,* vol. 18, no. 6 (November/December 1994), pp. 00–00.

Zoldbrod, Aline P. *Men, Women and Infertility.* Macmillan Publishing/Lexington Books, New York, 1993.

Appendix I   Self-Help Guide

Benson, Herbert and Miriam Klipper. *The Relaxation Response.* Avon Books, New York, 1995.

Benson, Herbert and Eileen M. Stuart. *The Wellness Book.* Birch Lane Press, Carol Publishing Group, New York, 1992.

Borysenko, Joan. *Minding the Body, Mending the Mind.* Bantam Books, New York, 1988.

Domar, Alice, and Henry Dreher. *Healthy Mind, Healthy Woman: Using the Mind-Body Connection to Manage Stress and Take Control of Your Life.* Henry Holt, New York, 1996.

Naparstek, Belleruth. *Staying Well with Guided Imagery.* Warner Books, New York, 1994.

Kabat-Zinn, Jon. *Full Catastrophe Living: Using the Wisdom of Your Body and Mind to Face Stress, Pain and Illness.* Delacorte Press, New York, 1991.

Zoldbrod, Aline P. *Getting Around the Boulder in the Road: Using Imagery to Cope with Fertility Problems.* Center for Reproductive Problems, Lexington, Mass., 1990.

PERMISSIONS

INDEX